Healing Herbs and Home Remedies-1

Healing Herbs and Home Remedies-1

Dr. Sukhram Khangarani

RAHI PRAKASHAN
Delhi-110053

ISBN : 978-93-80208-86-2

Publisher
Rahi Prakashan
L-45, Gali no. 5, Kartar Nagar
Delhi-110053

1st Edition
2024

Price
1095 /-

Type Setting
D. C. Computer, Ghaziabad

Printers
Shiv Shakti Printers, Delhi-110032

Healing Herbs and Home Remedies-1 *By* (in English)

By Dr. Sukhram Khangarani

Contents

Introduction

For thousands of years, in ancient India, China and in other countries, remedies from medicinal plants have cured a lot of people from all kinds of diseases. Herbal remedies also usually do not cause any side effects. Tradition of medicinal plants use in India is about 4000 years old. In the Ayurveda, about 1400 plants are documented in various texts. In Charaka Samhita, Sushruta Samhita and Ashtang Hridaya we can find more than 600 plants. Rig Veda (4500 to about 1600 BC) is perhaps the oldest document where medicinal plants have been described. Atharva Veda, also describes medicinal uses of large number of plants. Another treatise Dravya Guna Shastra provides information about medicinal plants from pharmacological point of view. Similarly, Unani and other systems of medicine practiced in India are largely dependent on medicinal plants. The wider acceptance of herbal based formulations is the growing recognition that natural products are non-narcotic and almost without side effects.

The Indian systems of treatment lay adequate stress on balanced diet and on inclusion of specific items in food to provide immunity against diseases. Also, number of plants products with medicinal properties form constituents of food. Even spices are being found to have medicinal properties. For example, capsicum, garlic, turmeric, onion, ginger, black pepper, cinnamon, curry leaf etc. have been found to protect against various health problems as well provide cure from certain diseases. Tamarind is used in curries, chutneys, sauces etc. as spice. Its unripe fruit is used for seasoning of food. Its pulp is rich in iron, calcium, potassium, phosphorous, riboflavin, thiamine, niacin, carbohydrates, fiber, invert sugar etc.

Vitamin C is present in substantial quantity in green fruits. Amla has been used as such or for 'chutney', pickle, 'murabba' etc. 'Charaka Samhita' records it as the most potent rejuvenating agent. Modern studies have proved that amla is extremely rich in vitamin C and Pectin, containing more than 150 times vitamin C compared to apple. Amla is an effective anti-ageing agent. It replaces worn out tissues with new ones. Contribution made by the Indian systems of medicines and folk traditions have been acknowledged by the WHO (World Health Organization) as well.

India has about 15000 species of medicinal plants. Presently about 8000 of these are in use as follows: Ayurveda 1769 species, Siddha - 1121 species , Unani - 751 species Amchi or Tibetan 279, Folk - 4671 species India ranks second in the world after China in export of medicinal plants. The global trade of medicinal plants stands at $7,592 million in 2011, and of these China and India's share was around $1,329 million and $790 million respectively, Anil Kumar, secretary (AYUSH), told reporters. India has registered a growth of 137 percent in export of medicinal plants in global market from Rs.554 crore in 2005-06 to Rs.1,318 crore.

Medicinal plants based industry in the country has an annual turn over of about Rs.42,000/- million per year and it is estimated to grow at the rate of about 20 per cent per year. There are hundreds of manufacturers and exporters in the country who are benefiting and large number of people is getting direct and indirect employment in these activities. About 800 to 900 medicinal plants are in all India trade, about 700 are obtained from the forests and many of these are harvested in large quantities. Common examples are neem, sena, amla, asoka, harra, gulancha, khas, ashwagandha, sarpgandha etc. Due to excessive and unscientific harvesting, large numbers of medicinal plant species are under threat.

There are approximately 1250 Indian medicinal plants which are used in formulating therapeutic preparations used in traditional systems of medicine. Recent surveys have shown that the percentage of natural products in the modern drug armamentarium is fairly high and is estimated to be varying from 35 per cent to 50 per cent. Almost every class of drug includes a model structure derived from nature, exhibiting the classical effect of that specific harmacological category.

Medicinal herbs can be used in many ways: dried and decocted as tea, infused in alcohol as a tincture, steeped in vinegar or honey. Herbs can also be steeped in oil and rubbed into the body for healing. When medicinal herbs are steeped in oil their healing qualities are infused into the oil. They are absorbed into the body through the skin. Oils created with St. John's Wort, Calendula and Plantain can be used to soothe muscles, heal the skin and take away itchiness.

In modern times too, people are increasingly turning to medicinal herbs as a source of alternative therapy. One of the major benefits of medicinal herbs is that they have no major side effects. They differ from synthetically manufactured compounds in that they are composed of ingredients that work together to produce a synergistic effect. However, these ingredients are quite strong and should be taken in moderate amounts, as excessive use of these compounds can have hazardous effects on human health. Also, these compounds can interfere and interact with certain drugs, if taken at the same time. Hence, extreme caution should be employed while using herbs to cure medical ailments.

Introduction to Home Remedies

Every country has traditional cures for its diseases. From homely recipes to complicated modes of treatment are found to have evolved, depending on the geographical position of the country, its culture, minerals resources and such other factors. Through the age India's myriad herbs, spices and plants have played a great role in the accumulation of ancient medical knowledge. By observation, experience and trail, the ancients came to posses an intimate knowledge of the properties of our plants life. We have been drawn to traditional methods of treatment for numbers of years.

It used to fascinate us grandma suggest a turmeric and chuna liniment for a sprained ankle, adadoda decoction to cure a cough or mulathi infusion for early rheumatism. This interest has been growing steadily since decades we have ample opportunity to collect first hand information from various sources. No side effects will be occurring by using any of the treatment described here. Basic ingredients used are easily available in nearest market. This home remedies are advocated by Vaids and Hakims with their rigid dietic restriction have been excluded as well as medical practices based on occult beliefs. Any lay person could easily prepare the remedies prescribed here at home before resorting to more sophisticated, complex, modern therapy. Actually most of minor ailments require to be treated only with simple home remedies and for most common ailments simple home remedies are available.

Many of these remedies are still in use in rural India. These in fact form the basis of health care in greater party of India. In some remote areas, home remedies of elderly females in the family is all that is available by the way of medical help. And often the treatment works; cures is complete. Only when disease get

complicated and goes beyond the ability at that time this home remedies do a needful work.

Most of the home remedies are not measured precise but the ingredients used are harmless a little more or less does not really matters. Home remedies have great advantages that they help the body mechanisms to fight disease unlike modern medicines which, without waiting for the body defence to tackle the problem, directly and in the process greatly weaken the system.

The modern urbanite, from infancy through adulthood to old age subjected to continuous chemical bombarding. Whether due to the use of artificial manures, disinfection of land, water and vegetation with the chemical pesticides or the excessive ingestion of synthetic man-made drugs as tonics and medicines, the human system gets saturated with chemicals. Without resorting to retrograde steps one should try to minimize this influence. At least in the field of health care, home remedies can check unnecessary synthetic drugging.

The idea of this book is to reach simple Indian home remedies to our urban homes where, alienated from traditional practices, patients are often drugged and even over drugged for the most trivial of health problems. Partly due to the patient's impatience and party due to the utter callousness of commercial medicines.

In the present times, natural cure home remedies are gaining momentum. Many people are heading their way towards adopting home remedy treatment to get rid of several forms of diseases. There is a natural home remedy for almost every ailment. The best part about them is that, they have no side effects and are absolutely inexpensive. Thus, not only are they safe for health, but also turn out to be an economical option.

Home remedy treatment makes use of things bestowed on us by nature like fruits, vegetables and herbs.

The Indian systems of treatment lay adequate stress on balanced diet and on inclusion of specific items in food to provide immunity against diseases. Also, number of plants products with medicinal properties form constituents of food. Even spices are being found to have medicinal properties. For example, capsicum, garlic, turmeric, onion, ginger, black pepper, cinnamon, curry leaf etc. have been found to protect against various health problems as well provide cure from certain diseases. Tamarind is used in curries, chutneys, sauces etc. as spice. Its unripe fruit is used for seasoning of food. Its pulp is rich in iron, calcium, potassium, phosphorous, riboflavin, thiamine, niacin, carbohydrates, fiber, invert sugar etc.

Vitamin C is present in substantial quantity in green fruits. Amla has been used as such or for 'chutney', pickle, 'murabba' etc. 'Charaka Samhita' records it as the most potent rejuvenating agent. Modern studies have proved that amla is extremely rich in vitamin C and Pectin, containing more than 150 times vitamin C compared to apple. Amla is an effective anti-ageing agent. It replaces worn out tissues with new ones. Contribution made by the Indian systems of medicines and folk traditions have been acknowledged by the WHO (World Health Organization) as well.

India has about 15000 species of medicinal plants. Presently about 8000 of these are in use as follows: Ayurveda 1769 species, Siddha - 1121 species , Unani - 751 species Amchi or Tibetan 279, Folk - 4671 species India ranks second in the world after China in export of medicinal plants. The global trade of medicinal plants stands at $7,592 million in 2011, and of these China and India's share was around $1,329 million and $790 million respectively, Anil Kumar, secretary (AYUSH), told reporters. India has registered a growth of 137 percent in export of medicinal plants in global market from Rs.554 crore in 2005-06 to Rs.1,318 crore.

Medicinal plants based industry in the country has an annual turn over of about Rs.42,000/- million per year and it is estimated to grow at the rate of about 20 per cent per year. There are hundreds of manufacturers and exporters in the country who are benefiting and large number of people is getting direct and indirect employment in these activities. About 800 to 900 medicinal plants are in all India trade, about 700 are obtained from the forests and many of these are harvested in large quantities. Common examples are neem, sena, amla, asoka, harra, gulancha, khas, ashwagandha, sarpgandha etc. Due to excessive and unscientific harvesting, large numbers of medicinal plant species are under threat.

There are approximately 1250 Indian medicinal plants which are used in formulating therapeutic preparations used in traditional systems of medicine. Recent surveys have shown that the percentage of natural products in the modern drug armamentarium is fairly high and is estimated to be varying from 35 per cent to 50 per cent. Almost every class of drug includes a model structure derived from nature, exhibiting the classical effect of that specific harmacological category.

Medicinal herbs can be used in many ways: dried and decocted as tea, infused in alcohol as a tincture, steeped in vinegar or honey. Herbs can also be steeped in oil and rubbed into the body for healing. When medicinal herbs are steeped in oil their healing qualities are infused into the oil. They are absorbed into the body through the skin. Oils created with St. John's Wort, Calendula and Plantain can be used to soothe muscles, heal the skin and take away itchiness.

In modern times too, people are increasingly turning to medicinal herbs as a source of alternative therapy. One of the major benefits of medicinal herbs is that they have no major side effects. They differ from synthetically manufactured compounds in that they are composed of ingredients that work together to produce a synergistic effect. However, these ingredients are quite strong and should be taken in moderate amounts, as excessive use of these compounds can have hazardous effects on human health. Also, these compounds can interfere and interact with certain drugs, if taken at the same time. Hence, extreme caution should be employed while using herbs to cure medical ailments.

Introduction to Home Remedies

Every country has traditional cures for its diseases. From homely recipes to complicated modes of treatment are found to have evolved, depending on the geographical position of the country, its culture, minerals resources and such other factors. Through the age India's myriad herbs, spices and plants have played a great role in the accumulation of ancient medical knowledge. By observation, experience and trail, the ancients came to posses an intimate knowledge of the properties of our plants life. We have been drawn to traditional methods of treatment for numbers of years.

It used to fascinate us grandma suggest a turmeric and chuna liniment for a sprained ankle, adadoda decoction to cure a cough or mulathi infusion for early rheumatism. This interest has been growing steadily since decades we have ample opportunity to collect first hand information from various sources. No side effects will be occurring by using any of the treatment described here. Basic ingredients used are easily available in nearest market. This home remedies are advocated by Vaids and Hakims with their rigid dietic restriction have been excluded as well as medical practices based on occult beliefs. Any lay person could easily prepare the remedies prescribed here at home before resorting to more sophisticated, complex, modern therapy. Actually most of minor ailments require to be treated only with simple home remedies and for most common ailments simple home remedies are available.

Many of these remedies are still in use in rural India. These in fact form the basis of health care in greater party of India. In some remote areas, home remedies of elderly females in the family is all that is available by the way of medical help. And often the treatment works; cures is complete. Only when disease get

complicated and goes beyond the ability at that time this home remedies do a needful work.

Most of the home remedies are not measured precise but the ingredients used are harmless a little more or less does not really matters. Home remedies have great advantages that they help the body mechanisms to fight disease unlike modern medicines which, without waiting for the body defence to tackle the problem, directly and in the process greatly weaken the system.

The modern urbanite, from infancy through adulthood to

old age subjected to continuous chemical bombarding. Whether due to the use of artificial manures, disinfection of land, water and vegetation with the chemical pesticides or the excessive ingestion of synthetic man-made drugs as tonics and medicines, the human system gets saturated with chemicals. Without resorting to retrograde steps one should try to minimize this influence. At least in the field of health care, home remedies can check unnecessary synthetic drugging.

The idea of this book is to reach simple Indian home remedies to our urban homes where, alienated from traditional practices, patients are often drugged and even over drugged for the most trivial of health problems. Partly due to the patient's impatience and party due to the utter callousness of commercial medicines.

In the present times, natural cure home remedies are gaining momentum. Many people are heading their way towards adopting home remedy treatment to get rid of several forms of diseases. There is a natural home remedy for almost every ailment. The best part about them is that, they have no side effects and are absolutely inexpensive. Thus, not only are they safe for health, but also turn out to be an economical option.

Home remedy treatment makes use of things bestowed on us by nature like fruits, vegetables and herbs.

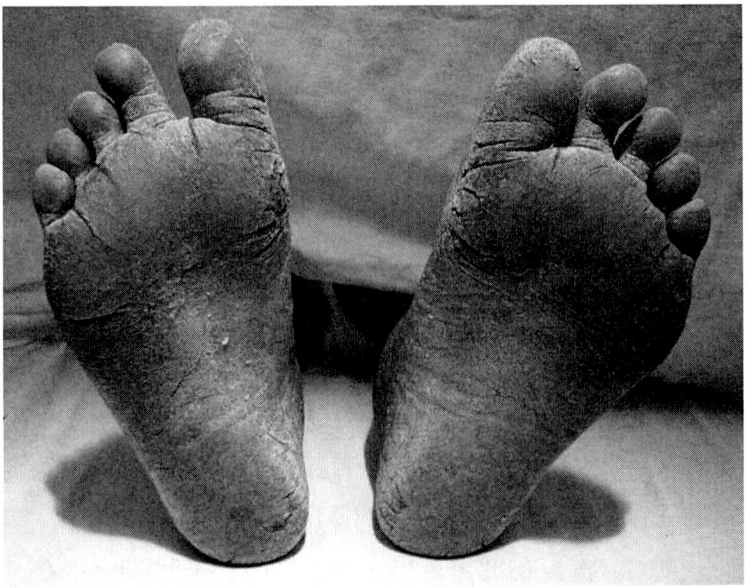

1. Athletes Foot

Athlete's foot is a contagious skin disease that affects the area between the toe fingers. It is mainly a fungal infection caused by the parasitic fungus dermatophytes. Medically known as tines pedis, the fungi live off dead skin cells and thrive in moist, warm places, such as gyms, locker rooms, showers and swimming pools. The symptoms of athletes' foot are burning sensation between toes, itching, redness, scaling and blistering. The infection is transmittable and can be caused by sharing the footwear of an infected person. Athlete's foot, however, is treatable and can be cured naturally as well.

Home Remedy for Athlete's Foot

- For athletes' foot, a simple home remedy would be a solution of one part vinegar and four parts warm water.

Soak the feet in this solution for half an hour, twice in a day.

- Baking soda paste would also be helpful in curing this infection. Take a 1 tbsp baking soda and add some water, to form a paste. Apply the paste on the affected area. Once dry, rinse off and let your feet dry.
- Add 40 drops of tea tree oil to a liter of water. Immerse your feet in this solution for about ten minutes. After this, dry your feet with a towel. Use a dryer to make sure that there is no moisture left in between the toes. After that, apply a few drops of tea tree oil in the infected region.
- Mix one part of pure apple cider vinegar with one part of warm water and soak the feet, in the solution, for about 20 minutes. Cleanse the feet both before and after immersing, using a gentle soap. After the treatment, ensure that the feet are completely dry. Follow this remedy two times a day, for 1-2 weeks, depending on the severity of the situation.
- Using boric acid, Epsom salt and vinegar would be an effective way of getting rid of the fungus. Take a large bowl and partially fill it with hot water. Add 1 cup vinegar, 1/4 cup Epsom salt and 3 tbsp boric acid. Make sure that boric acid has been whisked well. Soak your feet in the water for about 15 minutes and dry thoroughly.
- Apply cornstarch on your feet, including the area between the toes as well, before putting on socks and shoes. This will keep the feet dry and help in curing athlete's foot.
- Another efficient remedy would be to put fresh garlic slices in your shoes and wear them throughout the day.
- Dissolve 6 aspirins in 1/2 cup of rubbing alcohol. Shake the mixture well and apply on the affected area. Repeat this about thrice a day and continue it for three days or until athlete's foot is gone.

- Take a large bowl of warm water and soak your feet in it. Try to remove as much hard skin as possible. After this, pat dry your feet and apply a thin layer of oregano oil. Though it may emit a terrible smell, it is very effective in treating athlete's foot.

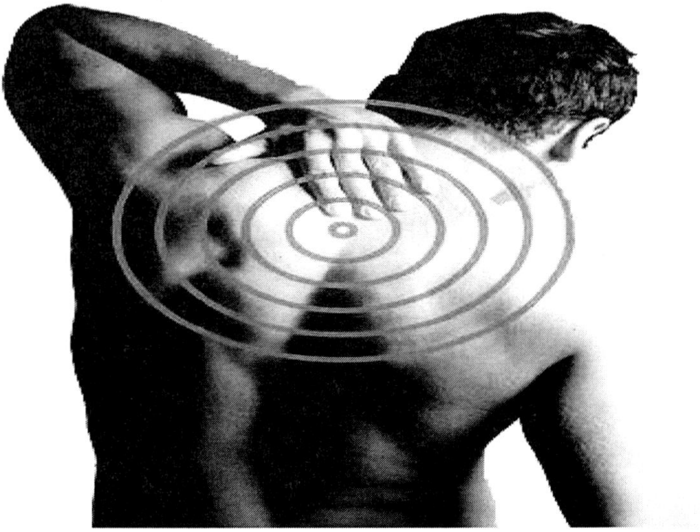

2. Backache

Backache, also known as lumbago, is one of the most widespread ailments found in people. It can be described as mild to sever pain in the lower back region of the sufferer. The pain may, at times, be excruciating and unbearable. Backache results in difficulty in bending forward, backward or even sideward. The problem is not restricted to older people and can also affect young people, especially those who indulge in a lot of physical work. Females usually face back during the pregnancy stage. The main causes for backache are strain, strained ligaments, back-muscle injury, excess lifting of heavy objects and disc disorders. Backache is a degenerative disorder but can be cured with the help of home remedies.

Home Remedy for Backache

- An effective home remedy for backache would comprise of a combination of wheat, Cuscus grass and coriander. Soak 60 grams wheat in water, overnight. The next morning, add 30 grams each of Cuscus grass and coriander to it. Add 250 ml milk. Put the mixture in a pan and boil it, until only 2/3rd of the quantity is left. Drink this concoction to get relief from backache.

- Mix 3 grams khas khas grass with 3 grams sugar candy. Take this mixture twice a day, with a glass of milk.
- Mix 1 tbsp glucose or honey in warm water and have it in the morning, on an empty stomach. It is a simple, yet effective way to get relief from backache.
- Eat two to three cloves of garlic in a day. Garlic oil can also be effective in curing backache. To prepare garlic oil, fry ten cloves of garlic in 60 ml of oil (mustard oil, sesame oil or coconut oil). Strain the oil, let it cool down a bit and massage the back with it.
- Mint oil has been found effective in curing backache. Lightly massage your back using some mint oil. It will give relief from the pain.
- Apply some heat to the back, using hot water bottle or infrared lamp. This would give instant relief from the pain.
- Massaging with turpentine oil is another effective home remedy for backache.
- An effective home remedy would be to apply potato, in the poultice form. Peel a potato and cut into cubes. Boil the cubes and mash them. After they cool down a bit, apply on the back and hold it there with a bandage, for an hour.
- Take out the juice of one lemon and add some common salt to it. Intake this, twice a day.
- Basil leaves can also cure a person suffering from backache. Take a cup of water and boil ten basil leaves in it. Let the water boil till only half the quantity is left. Cool down the water and add 1/4 tsp salt. Drink this decoction once a day.

- For tea drinkers, an easy remedy would be to add 5 black pepper corns, 5 cloves and 1 gram dry ginger powder to the tea. Have such a tea twice everyday.
- Include foods that have rich Vitamin C content, such as citrus fruit, tomatoes, blueberries and strawberries, in your diet.

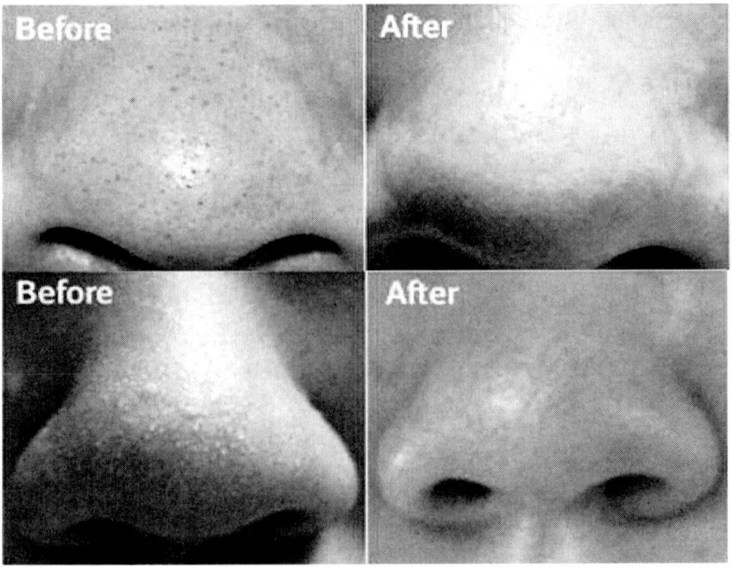

3. Blackheads

'Blackheads' is the name given to blackish bumps or plugs on the skin. They are nothing, but blocked pores that are filled with oil deposits and dead skin cells. A part of skin disease called acne; they usually appear on the face, back, chest and other parts of the body that have sebaceous glands. Blackheads are higher in number when compared pimples or zits. They thrive in oily skin and get worsened when the latter is exposed to pollution. You need to maintain proper hygiene to get cured of blackheads. While there are many skin treatments, like laser therapy, which you can follow to get cured of blackheads, it is advisable to stick to natural ways.

Home Remedy for Blackheads

- An effective home remedy for blackheads would be to combine hot water, Epsom salt and iodine. Put 1 tsp Epsom salt and 4 drops iodine in 1/4 cup hot water. When the solution cools down, apply it on the affected area, with a cotton ball. After it dries, remove it with a clean cloth.

- Make a paste of fresh methi (fenugreek) leaves, with water. Apply the paste on the affected area for about 10 to 15 minutes. Wash off with warm water. Use this remedy regularly for favorable results.
- For removing blackheads, taking steam would be beneficial, as steam opens the blocked pores. After taking steam, rub the affected region with a towel for 1-2 minutes. Thereafter, splash it with cold water, closing all the open pores.
- Another effective home remedy for blackhead removal comprises of a face wash, made of lime juice and milk. Add 1 tbsp fresh lime juice to a glass of boiled milk. Use this as a face wash regularly.
- Make a paste of ground radish seeds, along with water. Apply the paste on the affected area and rinse it off with water, when it dries.
- Yet another effective home remedy would be to make a paste of 5 gm red sandalwood and 5 gm turmeric, along with some milk. Apply this paste on the affected area and rinse off, after it dries.
- Mix almond powder with some rose water, to form a paste. Apply this paste on the affected area and keep it on till it dries. Thereafter, wash it off with warm water.
- Mix salt, lemon and honey, in equal quantities, and make a scrub. Yogurt can also be added to the mixture. Massage the affected area with this scrub for about 5 to 10 minutes. Rinse off and pat dry.
- Application of warm honey on the affected area, as a pack, would be beneficial. After the honey dries, wash the face with water.

- Combine equal amounts of groundnut oil and fresh lime juice. Apply this on the affected area and keep on for about 10 to 15 minutes. Wash off with warm water.
- Egg white can also be used as a home remedy for blackheads. Beat the white portion of the egg and apply on the affected area. Wash off with water. While wiping the area, scrub it lightly with the towel.
- Mix 3 tablespoons of honey and 1 tsp of cinnamon powder in a bowl. Apply this on the affected area and leave overnight. Wash off the next morning, with lukewarm water.

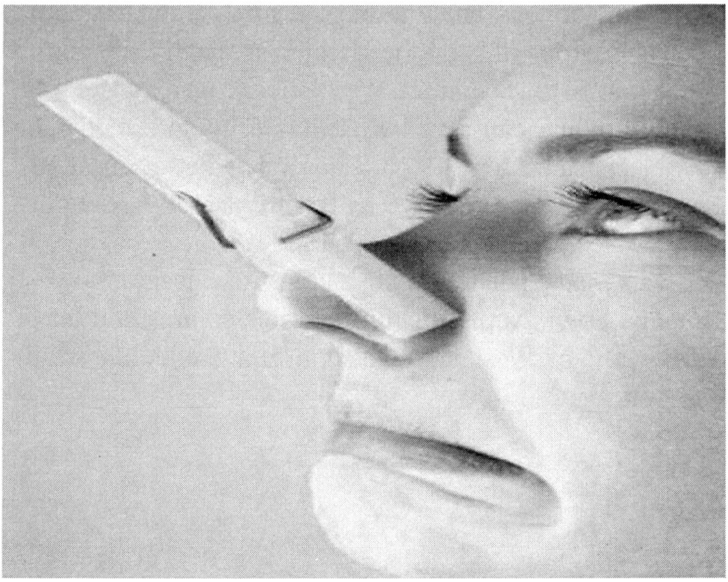

4. Body Odor

Body odor is the unpleasant smell which comes from a person's body, because of the bacteria growing on it. The notion amongst people that perspiration or sweating causes body odor is wrong. It may surprise you, but it is not perspiration that causes leads to body odor, but the bacteria that gets accumulated on the skin. The bacteria release unpleasant smelling chemicals, which, in turn, cause body odor. These bacteria multiply rapidly in the presence of sweat and this is why, people smell more when they perspire. Using deodorants only worsen the situation as it contains various toxic chemicals, which further aggravate the problem. However, the problem of body odor can be sorted out by resorting to home remedies.

Home Remedy for Body Odor

- To prevent body odor, drink a glass of water in the morning, on an empty stomach, along with 500 mg wheat grass. The chlorophyll present in the grass will help in reducing body odor.

- You can also apply baking soda to your armpits as well as to your feet, to reduce body odor.
- While bathing, add alcohol or white vinegar to a mug of water and use it to rinse the armpits. This will definitely help in lessening the body odor.
- One of the simple home remedies for body odor is to put a few drops of rose water in the bathtub, before taking bath. It will give you a long lasting freshness and serve as a good substitute for deodorant.
- To reduce the pH of the skin and eliminate armpit odor, one can use apple cider vinegar instead of deodorant. Put it in a mug of water and use it to rinse the armpits, while bathing.
- Take showers, at least thrice in a day, in the summer season, when one tends to sweat a lot.
- Prepare a homemade deodorant with the juice of about two dozen radishes and 1/4 teaspoon glycerin. Mix the liquids well and pour into a spray-top bottle. Spray this in the armpits to fight body odor. Remember to store it in fridge.
- During summers, you can apply the baby powder or talc to your armpits, in place of deodorants.
- Pour some white vinegar on a cotton ball and wipe your underarms with the cotton. While the vinegar smell would fade in some time, you would remain smell-free for the rest of the day.
- Mix two drops of the tea tree oil (essential oil) and one ounce of water. Pour this in a spray-top bottle and use as a deodorant. Since tea tree is an antibacterial herb, it would act favorably in preventing body odor.

- Mix 10 drops of the essential oil in 30 ml water. Apply this mixture on the armpits to reduce body odor.
- Turnip juice is also effective in removing body odor. Grate a turnip and squeeze the grated pieces to extract the juice. Apply this juice on your underarms.

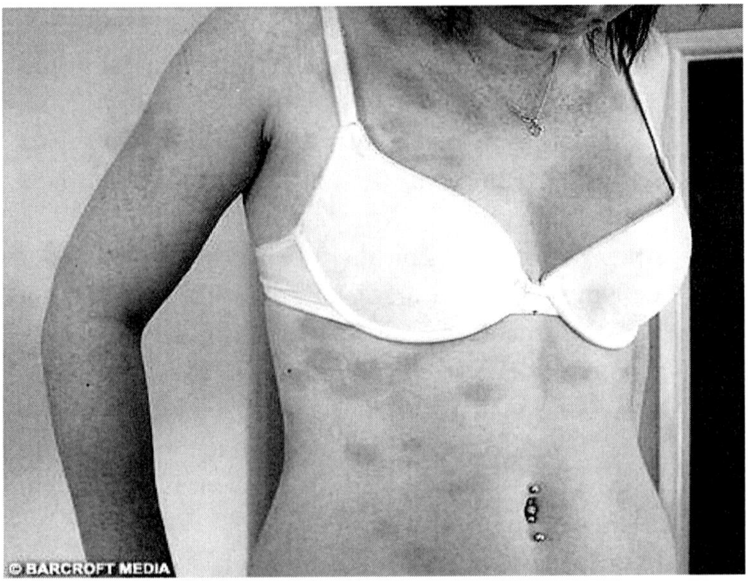

5. Body Rashes

Body rash is nothing, but an inflammation on the skin. Also known as skin rash, it causes a change in color and texture of the skin on the affected area. While some rashes appear on the whole body, a few occur on specific body parts only, such as back, face, neck, etc. The cause of body rashes might be a disease or an allergic reaction. While some body rashes are contagious, the others are not. Body rash is seen in the form of red, itchy or non-itchy bumps on the skin. There might be stinging or burning sensation over the affected area as well.

Home Remedy for Body Rashes

- An effective home remedy for healing body rash would be to wash the affected area with chamomile tea. Take a cup of boiling water and steep 2-3 tsp fresh or dried chamomile flowers in it. Strain the decoction and cool it down.

- Olive oil is said to have therapeutic qualities. Apply olive oil to the affected area. It would penetrate the skin and cure the rash.
- A simple way to treat body rash would be to apply Aloe vera gel or pulp. Apply this on the affected region. This would be very helpful in treating the body rash.
- Apply baking soda on the affected body part. After applying it, press the area gently. It would provide relief from the irritation and also cure the rash.
- A poultice made from yellow dock root, chaparral and dandelion would be effective in treating skin rashes. Take a handful of herb and blend in the mixer, with water, to form a puree. Apply on the affected area and cover with cheesecloth or bandage.
- Take a piece of cotton cloth and dip it in calcium water or comfrey. Place this cloth on the affected area. Not only would it be calming, but also help reduce inflammation.
- Blend 10-15 basil leaves with 1 tbsp olive oil, 2 garlic cloves, salt and pepper. Apply a coat of this mixture on the rashes.
- Increase the intake of food rich in Vitamin C. Citrus fruits will work best in this regard.
- Oatmeal bath proves useful in treating body rashes. Take a cup of uncooked oatmeal and pour it into the bathwater. Immerse your body in this water. Apart from providing instant relief, it would also heal the rash.

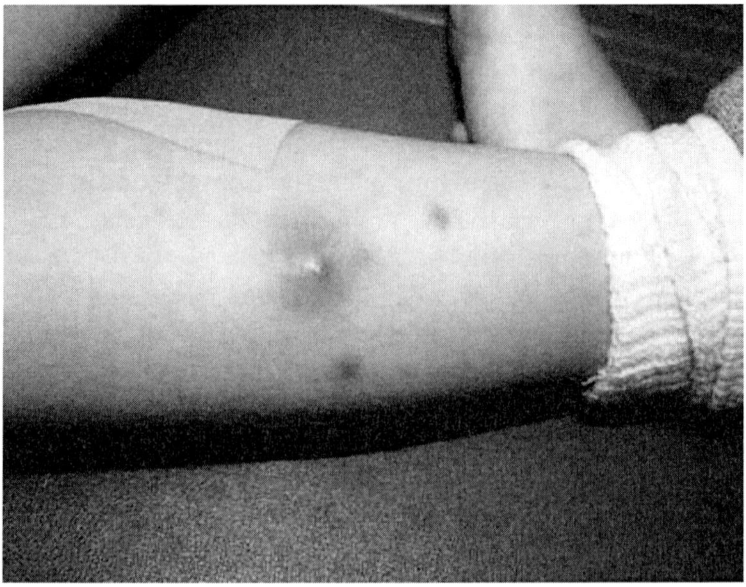

6. Boils

Boils are nothing, but a skin disease, caused by the infection of hair follicles. The problem is usually caused by Staphylococcus, a strain of bacterium that normally lives on the skin surface. While some boils which come and fade away on their own, without causing any trouble, others last a long time and cause pain and irritation. Face, shoulders, back, buttocks and underarms are the regions where boils usually occur. Boils do not come instantly. At first, the affected area becomes red and soft. There may be an itching sensation as well. Slowly, the boil begins to form. The bacteria that cause boils might also mix with the white blood cells, resulting in the formation of pus. Boils can be cured using some home remedies. Not only do they provide instant relief but also remove the boil completely.

Home Remedy for Boils

- Boils can be cured by using onions and garlic. Extract the juice of either of the two and apply it on the boil. It would ripen the boil and break it, thus evacuating the pus. You also use onion and garlic together, mixing the juices in equal quantities.

- For blood-filled boils, mix a cup of fresh bitter gourd juice with 1 teaspoon of lime juice. Have this mixture in the morning, on an empty stomach, till the boil gets cured completely.
- Another efficient remedy would be to apply a mixture of 1 tsp milk cream, 1 tsp vinegar and a pinch of turmeric powder, on the boils. This would ripen the boil without letting it get septic.
- Betel leaves is known for its medicinal properties. Gently warm betel leaves and coat them with castor oil. Spread the leaves on the boil and cover with a bandage. Change the leaves with new ones after every few hours.
- Make a paste of cumin seeds, along with water. Apply this paste on the boil and leave overnight.
- The decoction of margosa leaves is good for treating boils. Boil 15 gm margosa leaves in 500 ml water, until the solution reduces to 1/3rd. Apply it on the affected area, after it cools down.
- Hot parsley proves efficient in treating boils. Boil some water and steep parsley in it, till it becomes soft and juicy. Thereafter, wrap the parsley in a clean muslin or linen cloth and apply on the boils, as a poultice.
- Turmeric heals boils effectively. Roast a few dry roots of turmeric and dissolves the ashes in a cup of water. After five minutes, apply the solution over affected areas. This would ripen the boil and burst it.

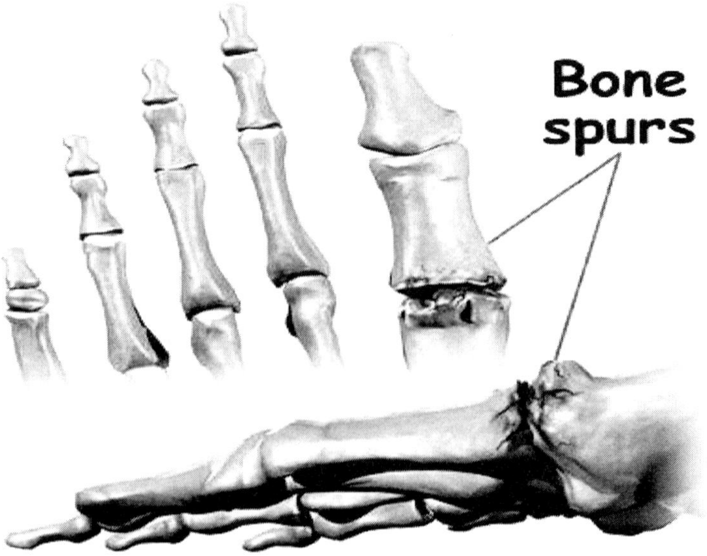

7. Bone Spur

Medically known as osteophytes, bone spur can be described as the growth of an extra bone over the normal bone. Bone spur is mostly seen in people who are above the age of 60. It mostly occurs along the joints, especially those of the spine, feet, shoulders, hips, hands and knees. While bone spur is not painful, it causes problem when it rubs against the normal bone or nerves. The condition of bone spur is indicative of spine degeneration, as it is caused when the surface area of joint is damaged. The most common symptoms of bone spur are pain in the back, neck, shoulder, thighs, arms or legs. There are some factors that increase the possibility of the occurrence of bone spur, such as lack of proper nutrition, faulty lifestyle, accidents and sport injuries. However, it can be effectively treated using some home remedies.

Home Remedy for Bone Spur

- To treat bone spur, the first step would be to lessen the inflammation. Applying an ice pack to the affected area would help reduce the swelling. Continue doing this 4 to 5 times a day.

- Another effective way to cure a person with bone spur would be to give him 500 to 1000 mg of curcumin (the yellow pigment of turmeric), 3 to 4 times a day, on an empty stomach.
- If there is pain, apply flaxseed hot pack to the affected area. Take a thick cloth and put heated flaxseed in it. Apply on the affected area and let it be there as long as it remains hot.
- Soak cheese cloth in warm linseed oil. Apply the cloth on the affected area. Cover it with plastic and keep a heating pad on the plastic covering for 2 hours.
- Indulging in alternate cold and hot water bath, for the affected area, would be effective in treating bone spur.
- Bathe the joints with chamomile tea. Take a cup of boiling water and steep 2-3 tsp fresh or dried chamomile flowers in it. Strain the decoction and cool it down. Use it to bathe the painful joints.

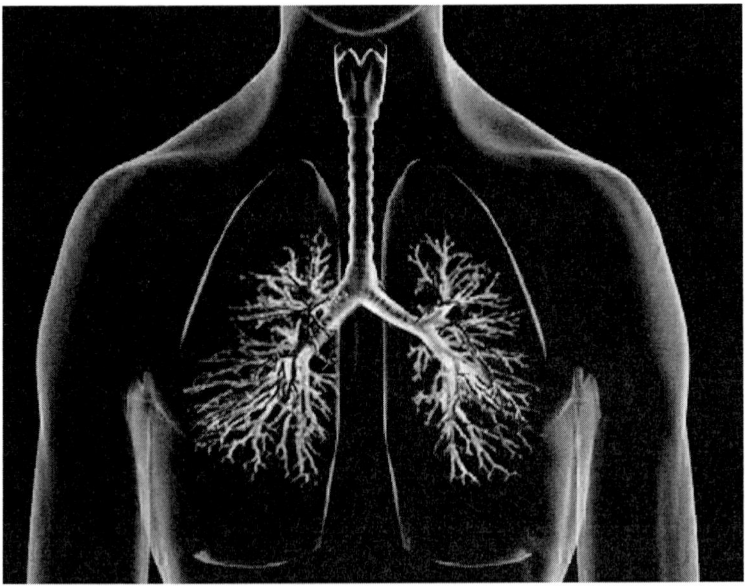

8. Bronchitis

Bronchitis is an inflammation of bronchi, the airway in the respiratory tract that carries air into the lungs. Its main symptom is a persistent cough that produces considerable quantities of phlegm. The other symptoms of bronchitis are coughing up extra mucus, wheezing and difficulty in breathing, apart from hoarseness, pain in the chest and loss of appetite. Bronchitis is usually classified into two types - acute bronchitis and chronic bronchitis. While the former is caused by viruses or bacteria and lasts for several days or weeks, the latter is a persistent, productive cough that lasts for at least three months and continues for two consecutive years. Mostly bronchitis is caused by an infection. Allergies and chemical irritations, such as atmospheric pollution and smoke of the cigarettes, are some other contributing factors. However, there are certain home remedies to cure a person of the ailment.

Home Remedy for Bronchitis

- The best way to cure bronchitis would be to consume turmeric powder. Put 1 tsp turmeric powder in half a glass of warm milk. Consuming this twice or thrice a day, on an empty stomach, would be beneficial.

- Mix half a teaspoon each of ginger powder, pepper powder and clove powder. Either mix them with 1 tbsp honey or put them in a cup of tea and consume.
- Onions have expectorant properties. Apart from liquefying phlegm, they also prevent its further formation. Intake of raw onion juice, early in the morning, would heal a person suffering from bronchitis.
- Mix 50 grams of fresh spinach leaves, 250 ml of water, a pinch of ammonium chloride and 1 tsp of honey and form a paste. Consumption of this mixture, on a daily basis, would relieve a person of bronchitis.
- Sesame seeds also have properties that can cure bronchitis. Combine a tsp of linseed, a pinch of common salt and a tsp of honey. Have this mixture before sleeping. It would help in the treatment of bronchitis.
- Another way of consuming sesame seeds is to powder half a tsp of it and mix it with 2 tsp of water. Have this two times a day. Yet another preparation would comprise of a decoction of half a teaspoon sesame seeds. Take it regularly, two times a day.
- Make a powder of seven almond kernels and mix it in a cup of orange or lemon juice. Have this emulsion regularly before sleeping. It would act beneficial in curing bronchitis
- Chicory is an herb that is believed to have medicinal properties to cure bronchitis. Grind the dry root of this herb and consume 1/2 tsp of powder, with one tsp of honey, thrice a day.
- Take some hot water, enough to convert one cup of linseed into a moist mealy mass. Wrap it in a thin cloth and apply this poultice on the front and back of the chest. Cover with a bandage.

- Another effective way to cure bronchitis would be to apply turpentine oil on the chest, every night.
- Castor oil can also act beneficially to cure bronchitis. Warm castor oil leaves on a pan. Let them cool down a bit, place them on the chest and keep overnight.
- Consuming fresh cabbage juice, on a daily basis, would be helpful in curing the problem of bronchitis.
- Steep half a tsp licorice root tea in a cup of hot water. After about ten minutes, strain the liquid and drink it, when still warm. Daily intake of this decoction, thrice a day, will show favorable results.

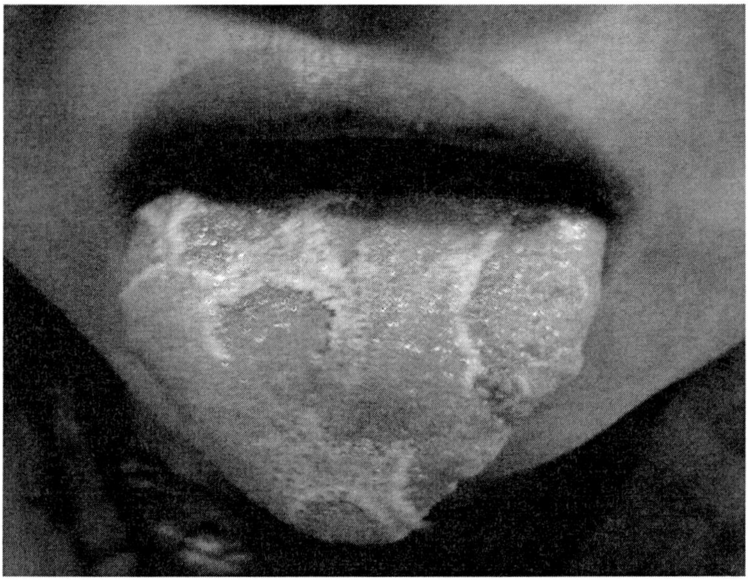

9. Burning Tongue

Burning mouth syndrome (BMS), popularly called burning tongue, is an ailment commonly found among people in the middle age group. While the exact cause of the ailment is not known, people suffering from it experience a burning sensation on their lips, gums, tongues, inside their cheeks, etc. Burning tongue can be acute, lasting for a few weeks, or chronic, lasting for months at a stretch. Some of the symptoms of this problem are dry/sore mouth, thirst, burning sensation in mouth, lips, palate, gums and tongue, loss of taste, numbness on the tip of the tongue and metallic or bitter taste in the mouth. The right kind of diet, combined with some conscious efforts, can cure a person suffering from this ailment.

Home Remedy for Burning Tongue

- An effective way to cure burning tongue is to suck on a piece of ice. It works wonders, treating the ailment effectively.

- Enhance the consumption of water. Larger quantity of water intake helps keep the mouth moist.
- Increase the consumption of food rich in Vitamin B, such as potatoes, bananas, lentils, chile peppers, tempeh, liver oil, liver, turkey, tuna, nutritional yeast (or brewer's yeast) and molasses.
- Apply glycerin on the tongue. It would give a cooling sensation, thereby relieving the pain and burning sensation.
- Another effective treatment for curing burning tongue is to have honey with milk. It increases the blood flow to the tongue, thereby healing it.
- For meals, resort to plain food, with lots of boiled vegetables. This would act beneficial in treating burning tongue.
- Lavender oil acts as an antiseptic. It not only works well to cure burning tongue, but also promotes blood circulation. Apply lavender oil on the affected area and leave overnight.
- Add iron rich food, such as broccoli, spinach and parsley, to your diet. They will help in treating burning tongue, by aiding the production of new red blood cells, replacing the damaged ones.
- It is recommended to have fresh fruit juice and vegetable juice, while suffering from burning tongue. These juices provide the necessary nutrients to the body and help relieve the burning sensation.
- Sugar free chewing gums would also be worthwhile in curing burning tongue. They keep the tongue moist and ease the pain.

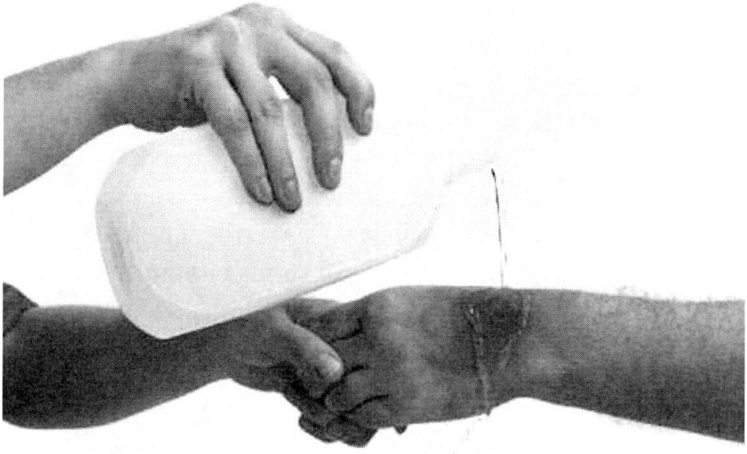

10. Burns

Burn is the name given to an injury that is caused by skin's exposure to excessive heat, electricity, chemicals, light, radiation, friction or fire. Most of us must have experienced the condition once in our lifetime. Burns can be categorized into three types - first degree, second degree and third degree, depending on the severity of the skin damage caused. While first degree burns cause damage to the top layer of the skin and get healed in a day or two, second degree burns are more severe and causes blisters. The latter are much more painful and also need special attention and care. Third degree burns cause damage to all the layers of the skin and are extremely painful. They make the skin look charred as the injury penetrates deep into the nerves.

Home Remedy for Burns

- The immediate remedy for burns would be to apply ice on the affected area. You can also dip the affected body part in chilled water, for about 15 to 20 minutes.

- The most popular and effective way to cure burns is to apply honey on the affected area and cover it with a bandage.
- Yogurt also acts efficiently in treating burns. Apply a generous amount of yogurt on the burn and keep it for about 15 minutes, before rinsing off. It would cool down the burnt area and provide relief.
- In case you have burnt the tip of your finger, tightly grip your ear lob. It might sound funny, but you would feel no pain at al.
- One of the effectual treatments of burns would be to cut a piece of onion and keep it over the burnt area. It would provide instant relief.
- Immerse the burnt portion in a bowl of whole milk for about 15-20 minutes. It would provide relief and cure the burn.
- Egg whites also prove beneficial in curing or treating burns. Beat the egg white lightly and apply on the affected area.
- You can also apply diluted vinegar on the burn. It would be very effective in healing the burns.
- Lavender oil also is helpful in treating burns. Dab the affected area with lavender oil. If the burn is severe, apply the oil 3-4 times in a day.
- Aloe Vera also treats burns effectively. Cut some fresh aloe Vera leaves and place them on the burnt area.
- After the burn gets healed, break a capsule of vitamin E and pour the liquid on the affected area. It would prevent formation of a scar.
- It might sound amusing, but applying some dish washing detergent on the burnt area helps ease the pain.
- Apply the papaya pulp on the affected area. The enzymes present in it would heal the wound and help remove dead cells as well.

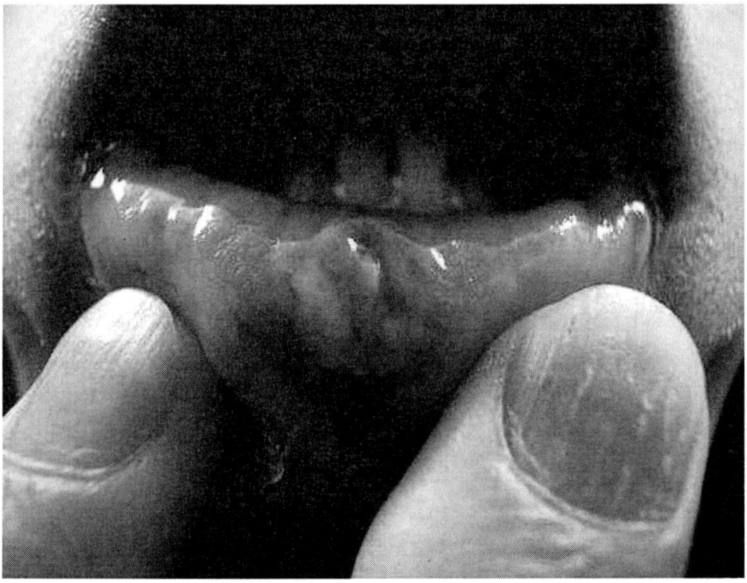

11. Canker Sores

Canker sores can be described as painful small ulcers, found inside the mouth or upper throat. These are white or yellowish in color and occur in the lining of the mouth, surrounded by redness. Also known as Aphthous Stomatitis and mouth ulcers, they cause much discomfort, especially while eating and talking. They are recurrent in nature and may reappear after being healed once. However, canker sores are not contagious do not spread from one person to the other. Canker sores appear due to various reasons - deficiency in nutrients, tension, stress, eating a particular type of food, indigestion, etc. They are not serious in nature and can be easily healed with the help of home remedies.

Home Remedy for Canker Sores

- An effective way for treating canker sores at home would be to apply raw onion on the ulcer.
- Aloe Vera juice, when used as a mouth wash, is beneficial in curing canker sores

- Another effective natural remedy would be to soak coriander leaves in water. After about 5 minutes, strain the water and use it as a mouthwash.
- Take a glass of lukewarm water and add 1/4 tsp cinnamon powder to it. Gargle with this water, first thing in the morning.
- Coat the ulcer with some honey. Let it stay for sometime and then salivate. It is one of the most useful remedy for treating mouth ulcers.
- Boil half a liter of water. Steep 2 tbsp Marjoram in it, for about 10 minutes. Strain the water and gargle with it, about 3 to 4 times a day.
- Gargling with salty water or barley tea is also found to be helpful in treating ulcers.
- Raw tehina, when coated on the ulcer, brings relief and cures the ailment completely.
- Increase the consumption of tomatoes and fresh papaya fruit. This is likely to bring relief and cure canker sores.
- Concentrated carob juice is also believed to be helpful in getting rid of mouth ulcers.
- When you have canker sores, it is advisable to brush teeth with baking soda, instead of toothpaste. This is because most of the toothpastes contain 'sodium laurel sulfate', which might alleviate the problem.
- Rinsing the mouth with Grapefruit seed extract would be helpful in treating mouth ulcers. Take a glass of lukewarm water and add 5 to 6 drops of Grapefruit seed extract in it. Use this as a mouthwash.
- Tea tree oil has medicinal properties and can help heal mouth ulcers. Apply tea tree oil to the sores, before going to bed, and leave overnight.
- Mix 1 tsp soda in a cup of warm water. Add a pinch of salt and gargle with this mixture, in the morning as well as before going to bed.

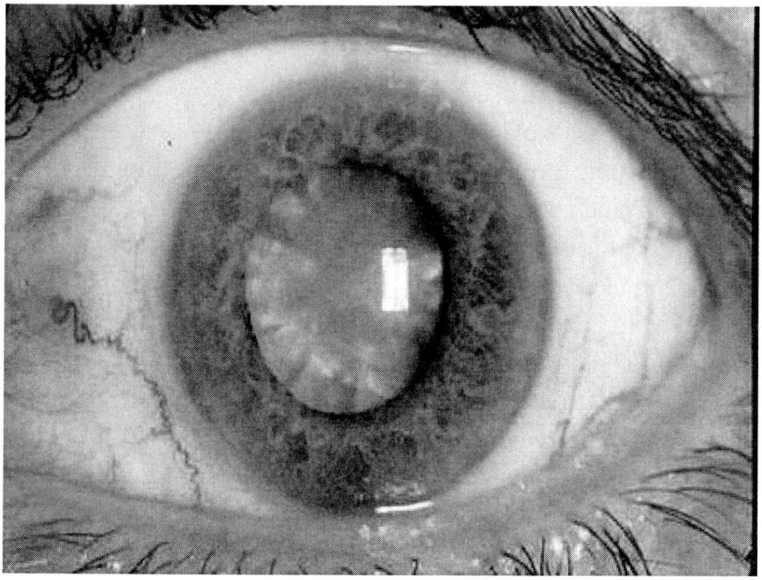

12. Cataract

Cataract is an eye disease which causes blurred vision. It results in the clouding of the crystalline lens of the eye, placed at the back of the iris, or in its envelope. The lens can suffer from slight to complete opacity, blocking the passage of light. A person suffering from cataract cannot see clearly. As the lens becomes opaque, it hampers the entrance of light which distorts the visibility. Cataract is mainly caused due to three factors - deterioration in the nutrition of the lens, deposits of acids and salts between the lens fibers, and disintegration of lens fibers. Aging, diabetes, eye injury and down-syndrome are some of the other causes of this disease. You can treat cataract naturally also, provided you know the correct home remedies for the same, some of which have been mentioned below.

Home Remedies for Cataract

- The most popular and efficient remedy for cataract would be to have carrots. Eat raw carrots regularly and also consume fresh carrot juice, twice a day.

- Another beneficial home remedy for cataract comprises of the extract or juice of pumpkin flowers. Apply this juice on the eyelids, two times a day, and keep on for fifteen minutes duration.
- Putting a few drops of honey into the eyes would act favorably in curing cataract.
- Aniseed is also helpful in treating cataract. Consume 6 grams of aniseed daily, in the morning as well as evening. For better results, mix equal amount of aniseed and coriander powder. Add a little brown sugar to the mixture. Eat 12 grams of this mixture, twice per day.
- An effective home remedy for cataract would comprise of almonds and pepper. Grind 7 almond kernels, along with ½ gram of pepper, in water and consume. Sugar candy can also be added to the mixture.
- A combination of cardamom and milk is said to be healthy for eyes. Grind 2 pieces of cardamom and put them in a glass of milk. Boil and bring it down to lukewarm temperature. Consume this milk, every night.
- Soak 3 to 4 almonds in 2 to 3 tbsp of milk and keep it overnight. In the morning, add sandalwood to this mixture. Apply this on the eyelids. It would reduce the redness associated with cataract.
- Include 2-3 cloves of garlic to your everyday diet, as garlic is known to cleanse the crystalline lens of the eye.
- Include oranges and grapes in your diet, as they help in healing the eye and curing cataract.
- Eat raw salads. Dressing them with olive oil and lemon juice would add to their benefit.
- Consumption of spinach, cauliflower, turnips, fenugreek, drum sticks, few nuts, soaked raisins, figs and dates is considered to be good for cataract.

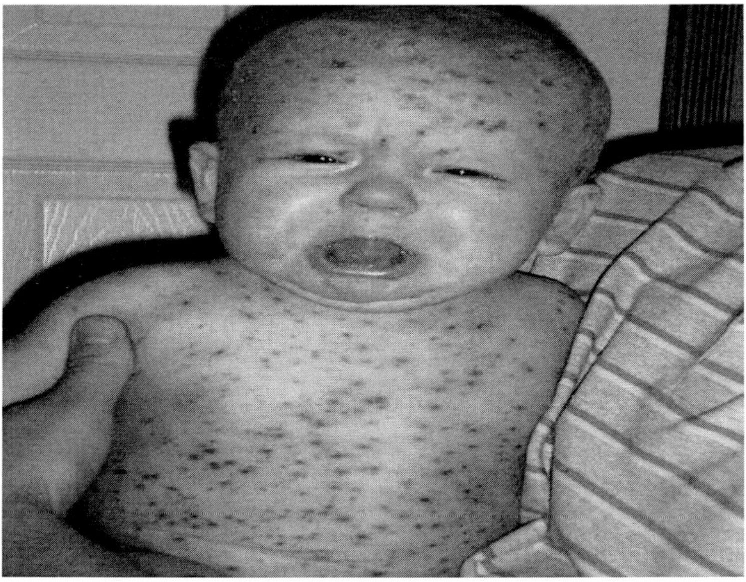

13. Chicken Pox

A highly contagious disease, chicken pox is a viral infection that is usually prevalent in small children, aged 3 to 4. Although the instances are few and far between, chicken pox can affect adults as well and in this case, it is much more severe than that in kids. Chicken pox can spread by direct contact or breathing in the air that has germs from an affected person's cough or sneeze. The most usual symptoms of chicken pox include low grade fever, mild headache, rash, loss of appetite and a feeling of weakness. It might be amusing, but the symptoms of chicken pos are not visible until it reaches the infectious stage. Vaccinations have reduced the instance of chicken pox, but the disease has not vanished altogether. Chicken pox is usually caused due to the virus called varicella-zoster. It might not be possible to completely cure chicken pox, as it would go on its own. However, the irritation and itching involved with it can be minimized, using some home remedies.

Home Remedy for Chicken Pox

- One of the most effective ways of treating chicken pox would be using brown vinegar. Add ½ cup vinegar to lukewarm bathwater. Apart from lessening the irritation, it would also help heal the lesions.

- Add 2 tbsp marigold flowers and 1 tsp hazel leaves in a cup of water and steep them overnight. In the morning, grind it and apply the mixture on the rash. It would help relieve the itching.
- Put a bowl of water in a pan and add green peas to it. Place it on flame and set it to boil. Once boiled, strain the water and apply it on the affected area. This would relieve the irritation and itching.
- Sandalwood oil also proves helpful in treating chicken pox. Apply the oil on the rashes right from the time chicken pox appears till its last days. It would also prevent scars from blemishing the skin.
- Coat the affected area with honey. It would not only relieve you of the irritation, but would also heal the rash.
- Grind oatmeal into a fine powder. Add 2 cups of this powder to the bath water. For better results, add one to one and a half cup of baking soda to the same water. It would help in healing the lesions
- Consumption of carrot and coriander soup would be beneficial in the treatment of chicken pox. Take about 100 grams of carrots and 60 grams of fresh coriander and finely chop them. Boil this mixture for a while. Strain the concoction, cool it down and drink it once a day.
- Immerse a handful of neem leaves in your bath water. It would provide healing effect and cure you of irritation.
- Application of Vitamin E oil on the rashes is another effective home remedy for chicken pox. Not only does it help prevent the itching, but also removes the scars quickly.
- Make a tea using chamomile, basil, marigold and lemon balm. Add a pinch of cinnamon, honey, and lemon to

enhance its healing property. Consuming this tea several times a day would be very beneficial.

- Mix 2 tbsp of queen of the meadow, 1 tsp of coltsfoot leaves and 2 tsp of marigold flowers in 2 cups of boiling water. After boiling the water for about 20 minutes, strain it. Cool the decoction and have it once a day.

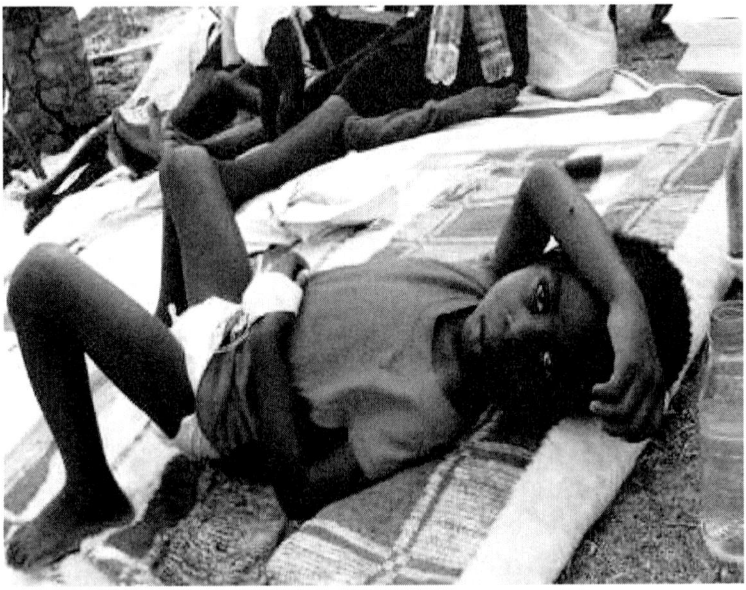

14. Cholera

A highly contagious disease, cholera is caused by bacterium Vibrio cholerae that affects the absorption of water in the small intestine. When it is severe, it causes diarrhea within a few hours, which means loss of fluid in a short spell of time. The loss of fluid would be through stools and violent vomiting. A water-borne disease, cholera can be prevented by taking caution over what a person eats and drinks. Drinking purified water and eating a healthy, hygienic nutritious diet would help you avoid the disease. There are a number of home remedies that can help cure a person of cholera, some of which have been mentioned below.

Home Remedy for Cholera

- The best way to deal with cholera naturally would be to have lots of water. It is very important to keep the body hydrated, so make sure that the intake of water is high. However, make sure to sterilize it before consumption.

- Onions are also beneficial in curing cholera. Take about 30 grams of onions and 7-10 black peppers. Grind this mixture and give it to the patient in 2 to 3 dose, per day.
- Cholera can also be treated by having a mix of water, sugar and salt. Take about 1 liter of boiled water and add 4 tsp of sugar and ½ tsp of salt. Intake this as many times as possible.
- Lemon juice and orange juice also act favorably in treating cholera. Consume at least one glass of fresh juice on a daily basis.
- Prepare a glass of fresh juice from cucumber leaves and mix it with a glass of coconut water. Consumption of this juice, in 30 to 60 ml doses, will relieve you off the disease.
- Another effective treatment would be to consume buttermilk. Add roasted cumin seeds powder and rock salt to it, for better results.
- Boil a few basil leaves in a glass of water. Strain the decoction, cool it down and have it once in a day.
- Mix 2 tsp each of bitter gourd juice and white onion juice. Once this solution is prepared, add a tsp of lemon juice. Consumption of this mixture two times daily would help treat cholera.
- Take three liters water and Add 4 gm of cloves to it. Boil this mixture until only half of it is left. Cool it down and consume it every few hours.
- A light diet would be efficient in treating cholera. Include rice flakes and corn flakes in your diet. Vegetable soup, with spices like black pepper, rock salt and ginger, will also be beneficial in treating cholera.
- Black herbal tea is also advantageous to treat cholera. Add ginger, black pepper, holy basil and mint to the tea and consume it at least once in a day.

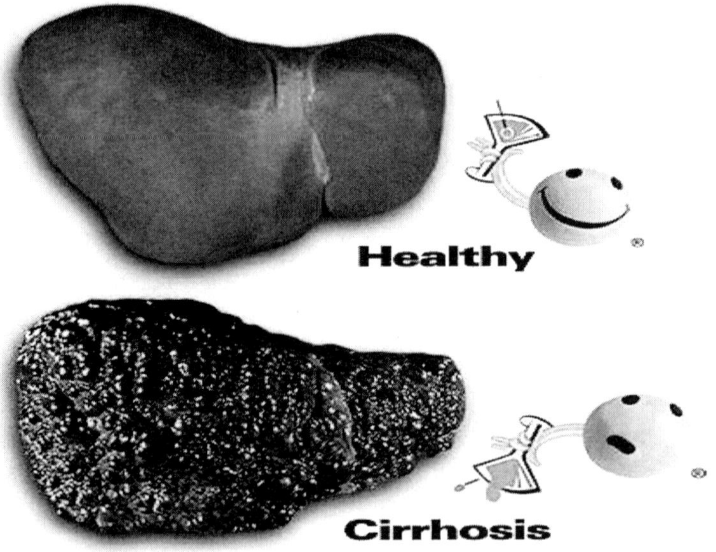

15. Cirrhosis of Liver

Cirrhosis of the liver may be defined in simple terminology as the contraction of the liver size becoming hard and leathery. There is a significant loss of cells in this condition – it not only injures the liver cells but also kills them. The most common symptoms of cirrhosis of the liver are frequent attacks of indigestion, occasional nausea and vomiting. Other symptoms include abdominal pain, low grade fever and foul breath. Liver cirrhosis may be caused due to excessive use of alcohol, highly toxic condition of the system and poor nutrition. The best way to cure cirrhosis of the liver would be to go the natural way.

Home Remedy for Cirrhosis of Liver

- One of the most popular and effective home remedy for cirrhosis of liver would be to have 200 ml of spinach juice. To enhance the efficiency of the drink add 300 ml of carrot juice to it.

- Papaya seeds also work effectively in curing liver cirrhosis. Grind some papaya seed. Once a powdery substance is formed, add 10 drops of lime juice. Intake this for about one to two times a day for about a month.
- Fig also proves beneficial in treating cirrhosis of liver. Rinse 4 leaves of sacred fig and crush them along with some sugar candy. Take this mixture and put it in a 250 ml of eater. Consume this mixture about twice a day.
- One tsp of glucose in a cup of water taken thrice a day would be beneficial in treating liver cirrhosis.
- Including carbohydrates in the diet would be helpful in curing liver cirrhosis. Salads also would be very helpful.
- Consumption of buttermilk with some roasted cumin seeds sprinkled over it is one of the easiest and effective treatments for liver cirrhosis.
- Another simple yet efficient treatment would be to have lime juice with a pinch of rock salt.
- Radish also cures a person suffering from cirrhosis of the liver. There are two ways of taking it. Either a person can take it raw along with the tender stem or make a juice out of it and have it empty stomach every day.
- Another effective way of curing cirrhosis would be to extract the juice of the herb eclipta. 1 tsp of its juice should be mixed with 1 tsp of honey and consumed three times a day.

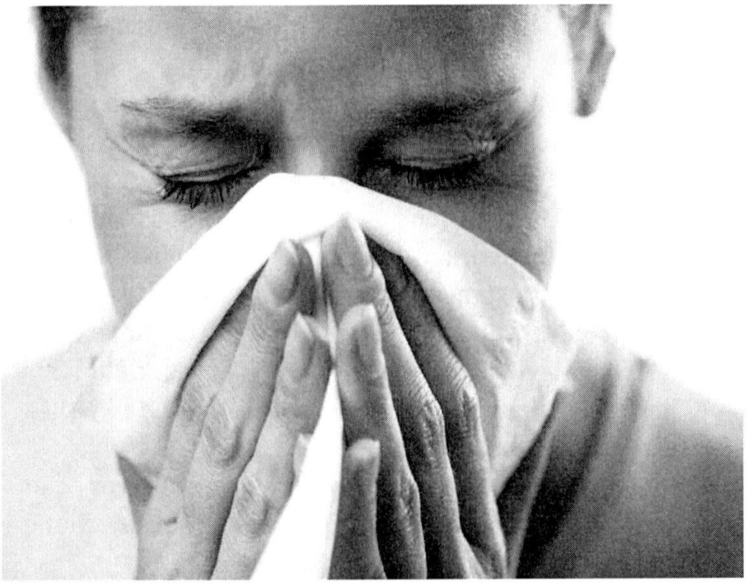

16. Common Cold

An inflammation in the upper respiratory tract caused due to viral infection is called common cold. The occurrence of this disease is very frequent and hence has been named common cold. Also known as acute coryza, common cold is not a one time disease and may appear and re-appear several times a year. It is most common though adults are also a victim of this disease. Common cold lasts for about 3 to 10 days and mostly affects the nose. Sometimes there is blockage in the ears as well. Bronchial tubes and sinus can also be affected. The symptoms of common cold are soreness of throat, congestion of nasal passages, running nose, sneezing, headache, chill and body ache. Common cold is not a serious disease and can be treated by adapting to some home remedies.

Home Remedy for Common Cold

- The most effective remedy for common cold would be to have lime juice. Take a glass of lukewarm water and dilute the lime juice in it. Add a tsp of honey to enhance its efficacy.

- The antiseptic properties of garlic make it one of the most effective ingredients for cold. Consumption of garlic soup would be the best way to cure common cold.
- Another effective method of using garlic would be to combine some garlic oil with onion juice. Dilute this with water and consume it for several times a day.
- Ginger also works favorably in treating common cold. Cut small pieces of ginger and put it in water. Boil this mixture. Once it simmers, strain the liquid and add half a tsp of sugar to it. Drink this hot.
- Hot water bath also proves effective as it relieves of all the nasal and chest congestion. Taking steam also would heal the congested nasal tissues.
- An excellent home remedy would be to have a glass of warm milk. Add 2 milligrams of roasted asafetida and drink this milk quite slowly two times in a day.
- Mix 200 grams of coriander seeds and jaggery in it. Make a paste of it and then add water in it. Boil this mixture and inhale the vapors of this mixture. Four times a day would cure common cold.
- Make a powdered mixture of black pepper and mix this in curd. Add jaggery or sugar candy to it. Take this two times a day to get cured of common cold.
- Take 250 grams of water and boil 7 pieces of each black pepper and sugar cubes. When the content comes to 1/4th quantity, stop boiling. Drink this mixture hot twice everyday to get relieved from common cold.
- Place 10grams of Sprague in a clean cloth and tie all the ends of the cloth. Apply indirect heat to it by keeping it in a vessel. Sniff this for a few minutes until it's hot. It would effectively cure nasal blockage.

- Mix equal amounts of tulsi seeds and ginger. Make a fine powdery mixture out of the two. Have this mixture two times a day.
- Cut 100gm lady's finger into small pieces and boil them in a liter of water. Once boiled, inhale the steam coming out of the decoction. Inhaling this one or two time a day would relieve a person from the irritation of the throat and the dry cough.

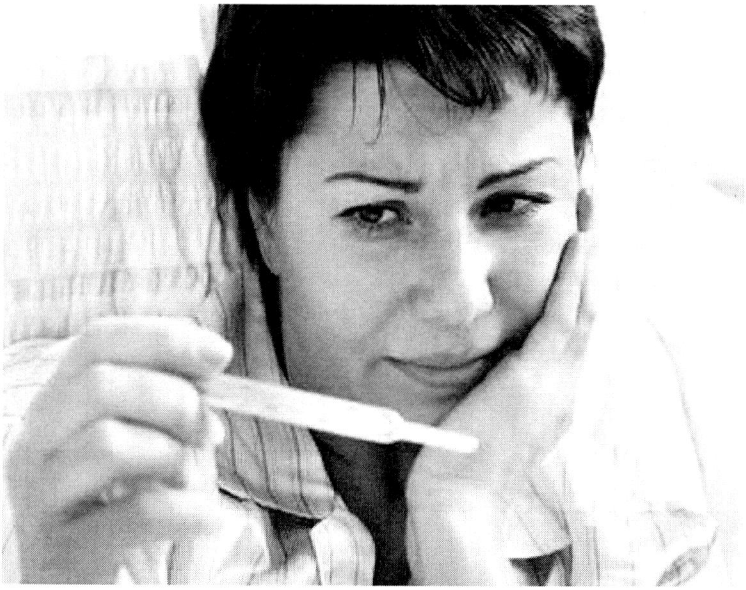

17. Common Fever

Human body has an optimum temperature range between 36.9 degree C and 37.5 degree C, or 98.4 Degree F and 99.5. Once the temperature goes beyond normal, the condition is called fever. There can be a little variation in the body temperature because of intake of food, the amount of exercise, and the temperature surrounding the atmosphere but once it exceeds this as well, it is a matter of concern. Fever occurs very frequently and is thus named common fever. In this ailment, the normal functioning of the body gets disrupted. The symptoms of common fever are rise in the temperature, profuse sweating, pulse and respiration becoming faster, slight shivering, pain in the head and body parts. Adhering to certain home remedies, common fever can be treated effectively.

Home Remedies for Common Fever

- The simplest and the most effective home remedy for common fever is to have a decoction of basil leaves. Take about 12 grams of basil leaves and boil them in half liter water. Intake this once a day to relieve from common fever.

- Saffron also works very well in treating common fever. Put half a tsp of saffron in 30ml of boiling water. After the water has been boiled, prepare tea out of it. Let the person suffering from it have a tsp of this tea after every hour.
- Prepare a tea using half a tsp of fenugreek seeds. It would not only providing a soothing effect but would also dissolves the mucus accumulated in the chest.
- Raisins are also effective in curing a person of common fever. Saturate 25 raisins in ½ cup of water. Once soaked, crush them in the same water. Strain the mixture and add ½ tsp of lime juice to it. Have this tonic two times a day.
- Add a tsp of glucose or honey to a fresh juice of apricot. Apart from reducing the fever, it also satiates the need for liquids and gets rid of harmful products.
- Grapefruit juice also acts favorably in curing common fever. Prepare ½ glass of grapefruit juice and add equal quantity of water to the concentrated mixture. Intake this mixture once a day to get relieved from the burning sensation.
- A person suffering from common fever is suggested to have lots of oranges. It increases the energy in the body and promotes resistance against infection.
- Another effective remedy to cure common fever would be to boil a cup of water. Add 1 tsp of turmeric powder, some ginger pieces, onion pieces, lemon grass, ½ a tsp of black pepper and 5-6 basil leaves. Intake this mixture three times a day to treat common fever.
- Mix 10 grams each of raisins and fresh ginger. Crush this mixture and immerse it in 200ml of water. After about an hour, boil this decoction until the quantity of the water reduces to 50ml. drink this decoction when warm. It would cure common fever effectively.

- Prepare a juice using the leaves of tamarind and some turmeric powder with cold water. Have this to eliminate infection and fever.
- Take 1 tablespoon of honey and add few drops of limejuice and ginger juice. Consume this mixture as it would effectively treat common fever.

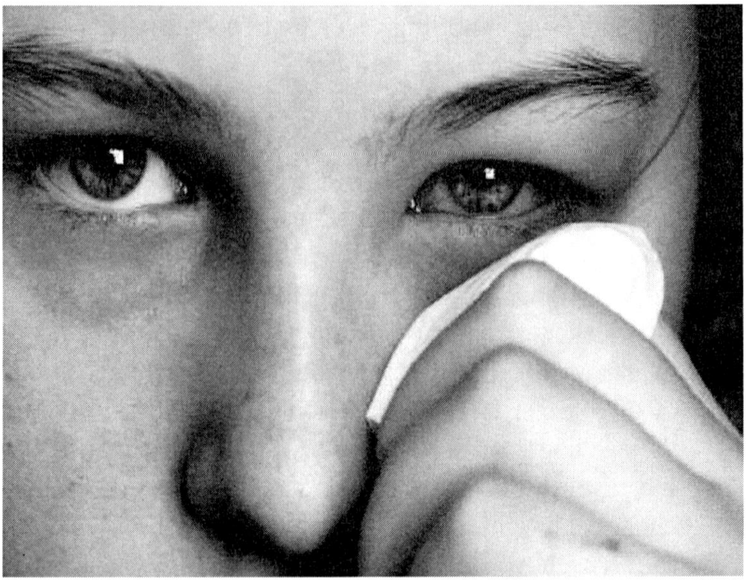

18. Conjunctivitis

A highly contagious disease, conjunctivitis is the swollenness or inflammation caused in the conjunctiva, a thin membrane which coats the front of the eyes. Also called 'pink eye' and 'eye flu', it is a condition when a person has sore eyes. Conjunctivitis is infectious and easily be transferable from one person to the other through direct contact. Symptoms for conjunctivitis are inflammation caused on the eyeball and underside of the eyelids. It also causes eye pain, burning, blured vision, feeling of dryness and discharge of a sticky fluid. On a severe stage, it also forms pus over and under the eyelid. The main cause of conjunctivitis is unhealthy and unhygienic state of living but since it is transferable, it may also be caused because of someone in the vicinity has it. However, it is treatable and can be cured using home remedies.

Home Remedy for Conjunctivitis

- One of the effective remedies for curing conjunctivitis is to mix 2 tsp. chamomile flowers and 1 tsp oregon grape root in 2 cups of boiling water. Once cooled, strain this mixture and use it as an eye wash.

- Sliced potatoes would also be beneficial in curing conjunctivitis. Peel the potato and cut it into thin slices. Apply on the affected area of the eye.
- Prepare a tea using goldthread leaves and use it as a eye wash. Not only does it cure the swollenness caused and the infection, it also relieves a person of the pain.
- An excellent eye wash for treating conjunctivitis would be to prepare a decoction using handful of dried coriander in 60 ml of water. It relieves a person of the pain and lessens the swelling as well.
- Increase in the consumption of vitamin A and B2 helps in curing conjunctivitis. The foods rich in Vitamin A are whole milk, yoghurt, butter, carrots, pumpkin, green leafy vegetables, tomatoes, mangoes, and papaya whereas green leafy vegetables, almonds, citrus fruits, bananas and tomatoes have high content of vitamin B2.
- Indian gooseberry juice has medicinal properties which cure conjunctivitis. Prepare a cup of this juice and add two teaspoons of honey. Consumption of this juice two times everyday would be beneficial.
- Carrot juice also is effective in treating conjunctivitis. To enhance the efficacy of this, add spinach to it. Mix 200 ml of spinach juice with 300 ml of carrot juice. Another combination of raw parsley juice 200ml, mixed with 300 ml of carrot juice also has therapeutic properties and provides relief.
- Sterile cotton ball and dip it in warm water. Use this to take away the crust formed on the eyelashes. Warmly compress the cotton against the eye to provide relief.
- Another remedy for conjunctivitis, would be apply poultice yogurt on the infected area of the eye. It would heal the itchiness caused.

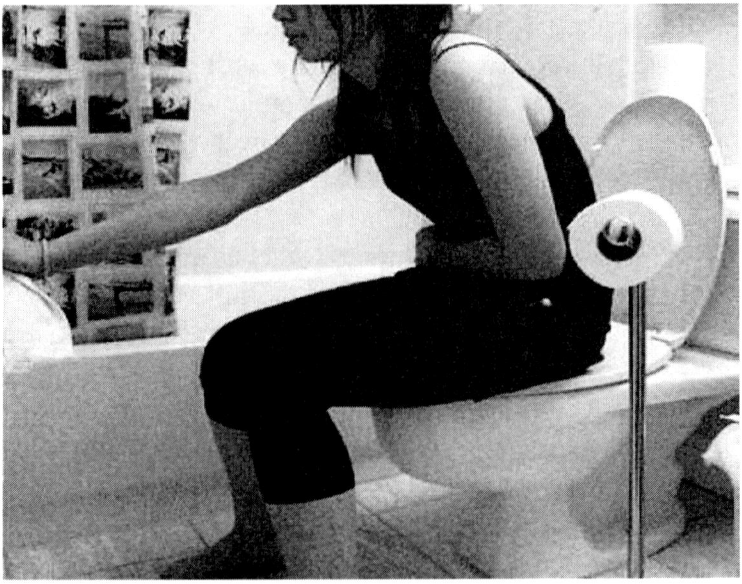

19. Constipation

Constipation is a problem of the digestive system. It gives rise to occasional bowel movement, incomplete evacuation of bowel, decrease in the volume or weight of the bowel. Not only is constipation a problem in itself, it is also the cause of many problems which occur due to it as toxins find their way into the bloodstream throughout the body. Some of the diseases caused due to it are appendicitis, rheumatism, arthritis, high blood pressure, cataract, and cancer. Some of the causes of constipation are low fiber diet, low intake of fluids, weak abdominal muscles and high intake of refined foods. When it comes to treating the ailment, the best way to do it is through the home remedies. Apart from solving the ailment, home remedies also add the required nutrients and have no side effect.

Home Remedy for Constipation

- The most simple and effective home remedy for curing constipation is to have at least 6 to 8 glasses of water. This is beneficial for digesting and dissolving the nutrients.

- Consuming 2 tablespoons of molasses before going to sleep is a good remedy for treating constipation. You can also add it to milk, fruit juice, or prune juice if you want.
- Cabbage juice also is beneficial in treating constipation. Have half cup cabbage juice two times a day to counter constipation problem.
- Immerse 10 to 12 dry grapes without seeds in milk and heat the milk till it boils. Strain the milk. While you are drinking the milk, chew the grapes side by side. It is one of the useful remedy for treating constipation naturally.
- An effective method would be to immerse 5-10 grams Spiegel seeds in 200 grams of warm milk. Add sugar to it and drink this before going to sleep. Another way of using Spiegel seeds would be to soak 2 tsp of them in water for about 6 hours. Add equal amount of sugar to the mixture. Before going to bed at night, have this mixture.
- Keep water in a copper vessel overnight. Have this water first thing in the morning in an empty stomach. It is a useful remedy for constipation.
- In ½ glass water, mix ¼ tsp of Epsom salt. Drink this combination to cure constipation.
- A combination of orange juice and olive oil would also act beneficial to cure constipation. In ½ cup orange juice, add equal amount of olive oil. Drink this to get rid of constipation.
- Mix equal quantities of carrot juice and spinach juice in a glass. Intake this combination at bedtime. It would cure constipation problem.
- A before meal technique would be to have a tsp of linseed with water. It brings in the much needed lubrication required for constipation.
- Consuming hot water with sour lime juice and half a teaspoon of salt added to it would be beneficial in treating constipation.

- Orange juice when taken empty stomach in the morning would be favorable in treating constipation.
- Fennel seeds will help to cure the digestive problem. In a glass of lukewarm water add a few fennel seeds. Drink this mixture every night before going to bed. It would definitely heal constipation.
- In case of chronic or severe constipation, have figs dipped in water. Consume this in large quantities in the morning time.
- A guava a day in the early morning, keeps constipation away.

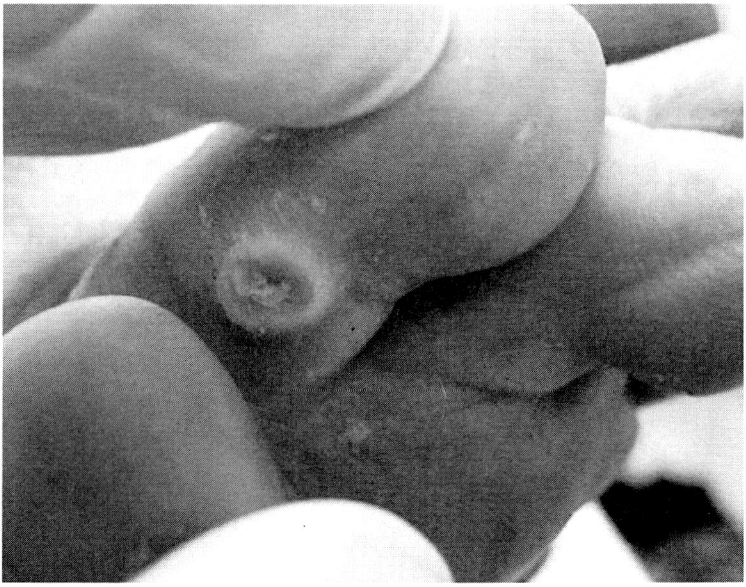

20. Corns

Corns are conical skin patches with its tip pointing into the foot. There are basically two types of corns - hard corns which are formed on the top of the toes or on the outsides of the little toes and soft corns, which are formed between the toes. Some of the causes of corns are wearing tight shoes, ill fitting socks, inflexible or nonporous shoes and high-heeled shoes. Thc most common symptoms of corns are pyramid like structure occurring over the joints of the toes and on the soles of the feet. However, corns can be treated successfully using a few home remedies.

Home Remedies for Corns

- An effective to cure corn would be to use lemon. Slice the lemon and place them over the corn, overnight. In the morning, remove it and wash the infected area with a disinfectant.

- Prepare a juice from raw papaya. Take ½ tsp of this juice and apply it over the hard area, three times a day. This will prove to be helpful in treating corns.
- The milky juice of the green figs also proves worthwhile in curing corns. For this, extract juice from the green figs. Take ½ tsp of this juice and apply it on the affected area, three times a day. Not only would it soften the skin but also prevent corns from occurrence.
- Increase in the intake of foods rich in vitamin and minerals would also act favorably in healing the corns. The person suffering from corns should go for a light and nutritious diet.
- Prepare a paste using chalk powder and water. Apply this paste over the hard area. This would be very effective in treating the corns.
- Indian squill has been effective in treating corns. The herb is made into a bulb like structure and tied over the affected area with the help of a bandage. Keeping this overnight would provide healing effects to the corns.
- Place a slice of onion on the corns and bandage them so that they are still. Keep them overnight and remove the next morning.
- Take a few ivy leaves and soak them in a bowl of vinegar overnight. The next morning, remove the leaves and dip a piece of bread in the same water. Apply this bread onto the corn and keep it throughout the day. Replace this with a fresh coat for the night.
- Dip a fresh cloth in rectified turpentine and wrap it around the area. Apply this several times a day.
- Dip a cotton ball with vinegar. Keep this until the area becomes soft. Once it is soft, rub it with a pumice stone.
- Tie the corns with a fresh pineapple peel. Leave it overnight. Regular use of this would cure the problem of corns.

- Boil some oatmeal in water for about 5 minutes. Strain away the water in a bucket and dip the corn affected foot into it. it would relieve of all the pain caused thereby healing the disease.
- The juice prepared from the stem of the dandelion also proves worthwhile in treating corns. Apply this juice on the corns for curing the disease.
- Add a drop of lemon juice into the brewer's yeast to make a paste. Apply this paste on the corn and keep it overnight. This is one of the most effective remedy for treating corns.

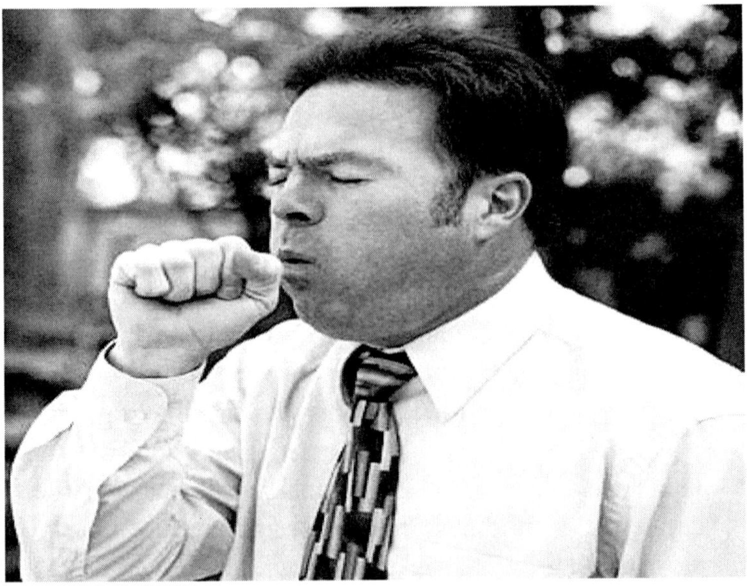

21. Cough

Coughing is a means by which the body throws out or gets rid of substances that are irritating the air passages in their way. Cough can be classified into two types - productive cough, which produces phlegm from the lungs and the other is nonproductive cough, which is dry and doesn't produce any phlegm from the lungs. Cough can be acute lasting for a few days to chronic, lasting for a few weeks. It is not restricted to any particular age group and can affect everyone. Coughing is accompanied with a typical noise from the act of exhaling air suddenly in order to clear the phlegm or the blocking. Cough can be treated at home.

Home Remedy for Cough

- An effective remedy for treating cough would to slightly cut a lemon and fill it with black pepper. Suck this as it would reduce the cough.

- One of the easiest methods would be to add a pinch of grounded white pepper in one tea spoon of pure honey. Intake this 2 to 3 times a day for about 4 to 5 days.
- Grapes tone up the lungs and act as expectorant. Increase in the consumption would be favorable in curing cough.
- Take 1-2 gm each of black pepper, long pepper, and dry ginger. Make a mixture of these ingredients and have it along with honey for 2-3 days.
- Increase in the consumption of garlic also acts beneficial in treating cough.
- Add ¼ teaspoon of red pepper, ¼ teaspoon of ground ginger, 1 table spoon of apple cider vinegar, 1 table spoon of honey in 2 tablespoon of normal water to make a paste. Make a paste of these ingredients and have it once a day for treating cough problem.
- Gargle with warm spinach juice. This is helpful in curing dry cough.
- For people suffering from dry cough, mix half spoon of Cuscus grass (khas khas) in 3-4 teaspoons of coconut milk. To enhance the efficacy, add one teaspoon of honey. Drink this before going to bed.
- Take 100 grams of raisins and grind it with some water. Add 100 grams of sugar and heat the mixture till it turns saucy. Intake about 20 grams of this every day before sleeping at night.
- Prepare a tea. Add aniseed and holy basil to it. Drink this tea at least twice a day to get relief from relief from cough.
- Soak almonds overnight. In the morning, remove their brown cover and make a paste adding 20gm of butter and sugar to it. Have this twice a day in the morning as well as in the evening.
- Another effective home remedy would be to chew 4 basil leaves and black pepper. It would provide instant relief and treat the cough quickly.

- Onions when mixed with honey also provide relief. Extract onion juice and mix it with honey. Consume this mixture 2-3 times' day. Another method would be to crush onions and add one lemon juice to it in a cup of boiling water. Pour in some honey and drink this mixture 2-3 times a day.
- Take 500 grams of water and Boil 10 grams of Sprague in it for 15 minutes. After it has cooled, add two pinches of salt. Gargle with this mixture two times a day. Apart from clearing excessive mucous, it would also soothe the throat.
- Boil a cup of water and put a 1 tsp of Marjoram in it. Leave this mixture for 10-15 minutes and then drink. Have this three to four times a day to get cured of cough.

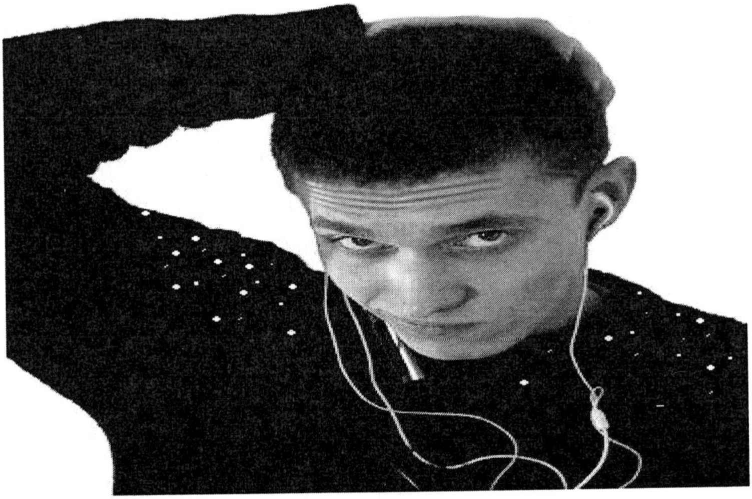

22. Dandruff

Dandruff is a condition wherein skin flakes come out of the scalp. These collect amidst the hair and sometimes settle on shoulders, face, eyebrows and clothes. There are basically two types of dandruff - dry dandruff and waxy dandruff. Dry dandruff causes itchiness. In this case the small flakes are loosely scattered in the hair as compared to the waxy dandruff which remains stuck to the scalp in patches. Dandruff is infectious in nature and can spread to others by using of common towels, combs, soaps and hairbrushes. The reasons for dandruff may be poor nutrition, deficiency of zinc, fungus or even high use of alkaline soaps and shampoos. Dandruff can be treated using natural remedies.

Home Remedy for Dandruff

- The best way to cure dandruff naturally is to have a hot steam bath. First, massage your head with hot oil and then wrap a hot damp towel. Keep this for a few minutes after which wash your hair.

- Take a small bowl of coconut oil and soak in it a few peels of lemon. Keep this for a span of 8-10 days. Strain the oil and apply this mixture on the hair.
- Combine two tablespoons of vinegar and six tablespoons of hot water. Take a cotton ball and apply the above made combination with it on the scalp. Keep this overnight and wash off your hair next morning.
- Take some beetroot juice and add a few drops of vinegar. Dab this on the scalp. Another combination would be to add a few drops of ginger juice in the beetroot juice.
- Another effective method to treat dandruff would be to combine 2 tablespoons of fresh apple juice with 2 tablespoons of warm water. Dab this on the hair and keep it for 10-15 minutes before rinsing. Do this for once or twice a week to cure dandruff.
- Mix olive oil and almond oil in equal proportions. Leave it for about 5 minutes. Once a burning sensation is felt, wash the hair.
- Immerse two tablespoons of fenugreek seeds in water overnight. Grind them the next morning to form a paste. Keep it for half an hour before washing it with a ritha solution or shikakai.
- Conditioning the hair using cider vinegar after shampooing also acts beneficial in removing dandruff.
- Heat 300 grams of coconut oil with 3 grams of black pepper. Strain this decoction. Once cooled, apply this decoct on the hair and the scalp overnight.
- Use a teaspoon of fresh lime juice as a conditioner. Apart from removing the dandruff, it also gives a glowing effect to the hair.
- For a person who applies henna, mash beetroot leaves in it. Apply this mixture on the head to prevent dandruff and hair fall.

- Washing the hair with green gram powder in curd twice a week would also cure a person from dandruff.
- Add two tablespoons of water to two beaten eggs and mix it properly. Apply this combination to the moist hair and leave it for 10-15 minutes. Rinse the hair with lukewarm water. This will be effective in treating dandruff.

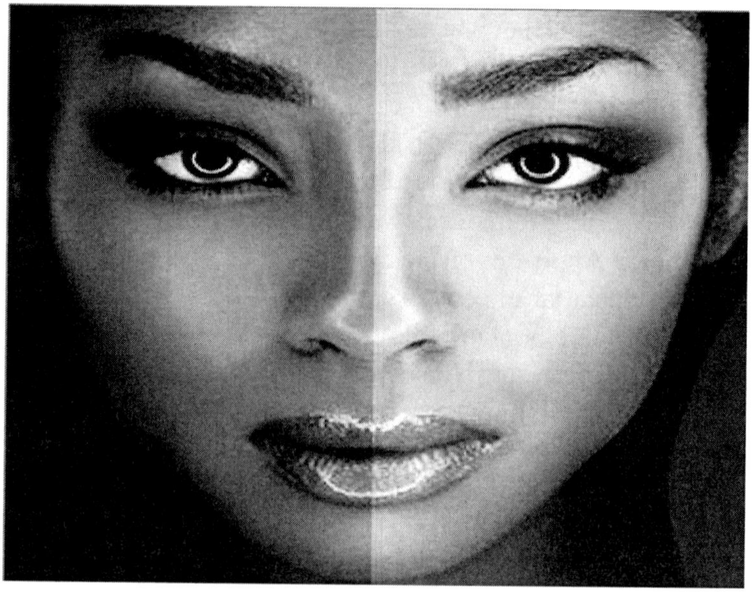

23. Dark Skin

While some people have dark skin from the time they are born, there are others who have it because of hyper pigmentation and various other reasons. Dark skin has higher quantity of skin pigment melanin, as compared to a fair skin. The increased quantity of melanin also makes the skin look blemished and patchy. The most common symptoms of dark skin are that the skin color turns to brownish to blackish. The effect magnifies if it is also accompanied with blemishes or dark patches on the skin. Dark skins can be cured naturally using some easy measures.

Home Remedy for Dark Skin

- An effective home remedy to cure the problem of dark skin would be to mix 1 tsp of milk powder, 1 tsp of honey, 1 tsp of lemon juice and ½ tsp of almond oil. Make a paste and apply this on the face. Apart from removing the tan, it would also make the skin shine.

- Take some oatmeal along with curd and tomato juice. Apply this mixture on the face and keep it for about 20 minutes. Wash your face with cold water.
- Potato acts as a very good bleaching agent. Slice a potato and keep them over the face. This would lighten the marks.
- Take a little turmeric powder and add a few drops of lime juice. Apply this on the darkened area. This would help to reduce tan effectively.
- Dry some orange peels. Then, mix them to a bowl of curd. This would be beneficial in removing tan. Keep this for about 15 minutes and wash off with cold water.
- Another effective remedy to remove tan would be to soak 4 almonds in water and keep it overnight. Grind these almonds to make a paste. Apply this paste at bedtime. In the morning, was off this paste with cold water.
- Take a tablespoon of gram flour and mix it with 2 tsp of raw milk and 2-3 drops of lime juice. Apply this mixture and leave it for 15 minutes before washing off.
- Mint leaves work well to remove the dark skin. Take some fresh ground mint leaves and make a paste of it. Keep it for 15 minutes and later rinse of.
- Grate a tomato and add 2-3 drops of lime to it. Apply this mixture on the face and keep it for 15 minutes. Repeat this two times a day for better results.
- It is advisable to increase in the intake of water. The more water you have the more toxins flush out from the body and hence have better glowing skin. As per the diet, include whole cereals, vegetables, fruits, pulses etc into your diet.

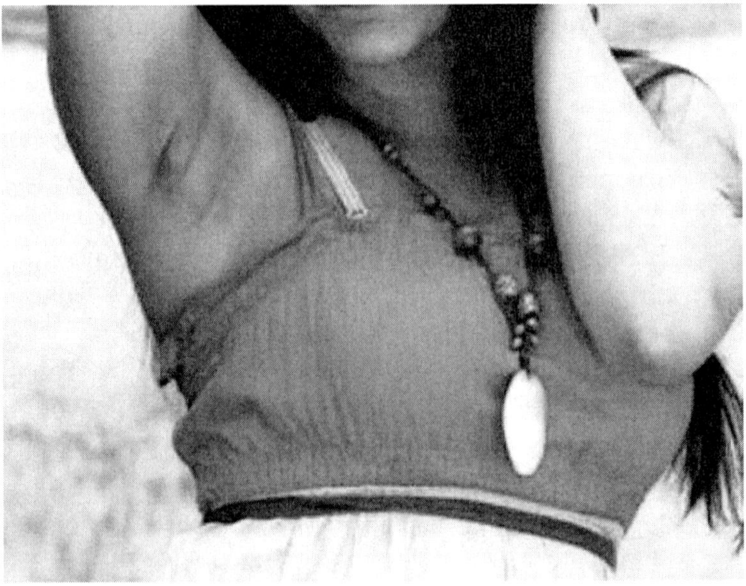

24. Dark Underarms

Dark underarms is a condition when the skin under the arms or the armpits as we know gets dark. Dark armpits restrict a person to wear sleeveless tops because it would be very embarrassing for her. Dark underarms can be the result of improper cleaning, sweating, dead skin cells and friction due to different types of clothes. For some people, it may be due to shaving products or deodorants containing alcohol. Dark underarms may be accompanied by itching, sweating and bad odor. There are several ways to treat the problem naturally.

Home Remedy for Dark Underarms

- The best and effective home remedy to treat dark underarms it to use lemon. Take a piece of lemon and rub it on the armpits.
- Baking soda also acts favorably in curing the darkness of the underarms. After bath, apply some baking soda onto the armpits.

- Apply Vitamin E oil on the armpits to treat dark underarms.
- Rub the underarms with coconut oil to remove the darkness from the underarms.
- Make a paste using 1 tsp of lime juice, 1 tsp of cucumber juice as well as a hint of turmeric powder. Apply this paste on your armpits and wash off after 20 minutes.
- Take 1 tsp of gram flour, 1 tsp of curd and a pinch of turmeric to make a paste. Apply this mixture to your armpits and rinse after it has dried with cold water.
- Mix a little sandalwood powder and a few drops of rose water to make a paste. Apply this paste onto your underarms.
- Potato is an active bleaching agent. Apply potato juice on the underarms and keep it for sometime. It would effectively remove the darkness of the armpits.

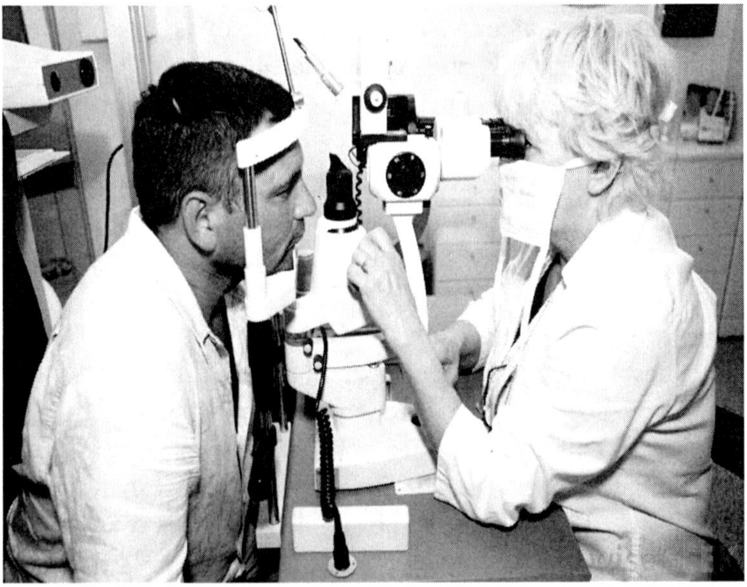

25. Defective Vision

Defective vision is the inability to see clearly. Defective vision may be of two types - myopia or short-sightedness. It refers to a condition when a person is unable to see far-off objects clearly. The other is hyperopia or long sightedness which is a situation when a person cannot focus and thus cannot see closer things properly. The blurred vision is also at times accompanied by itching and heaviness in the eyes. Also the patient may suffer from a mild headache. There are several causes for defective vision in a person. While some are due to external factors, the others may be internal. Though the problem may not be cured completely, using home remedies one can lighten the effect.

Home Remedy for Defective Vision

- The best remedy for treating defective vision is to increase the consumption of foods rich in Vitamin A. they are the best source for improving vision. Some of the food items include raw spinach, turnip tops, milk cream, cheese, butter, tomatoes, lettuce, cabbage, soya beans, green peas, fresh milk, oranges, and dates.

- Intake a lot of carrot juice as it has been found very effective in curing defective vision.
- Dissolve 30 grams of Triphala in ½ liter of water. There are two ways of using this water - one can either drink it or wash his/her eyes with it. it is an effective home remedy for defective vision.
- In a glass of milk, mix ½ teaspoon each of licorice root power and honey. Add ¼ part of ghee. Drink this milk as it would be beneficial in curing defective vision.
- In 200 ml of carrot juice, add150 ml of celery juice, 75 ml of endives juice, and 75 ml of parsley juice to make ½ liter of this juices. In this mixture, combine ½ liter of chicory juice as well. Intake of this juice everyday helps in improving vision.
- Sun gazing is also very effective in treating defective vision. Sit on the bench of the garden. Face the sun while closing your eyes. For ten minutes, shake your head several times. After this is done, open your eyes and blink about ten times while looking at the sun. it is also advisable to look at some landscapes. This would provide cooling effect to the eyes.
- One more method can be to splash cold water on the closed eye lids. Once enough water has been splashed, dab your eye with a clean towel.

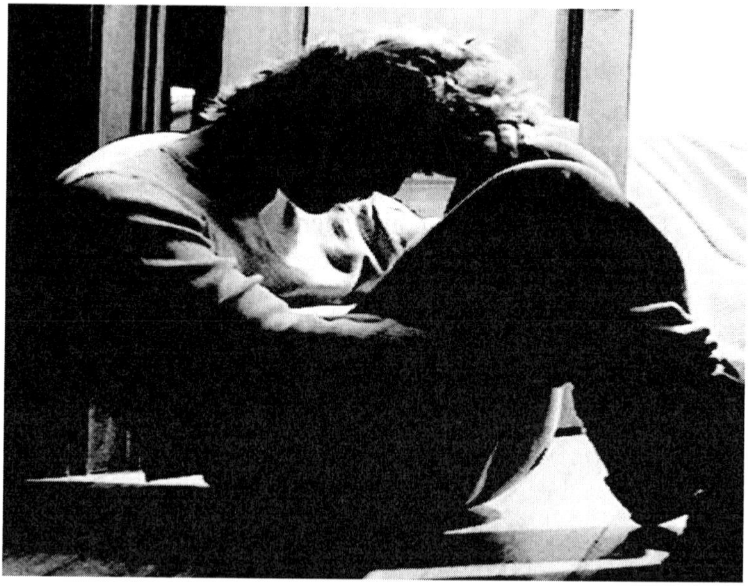

26. Depression

Depression is a state of the mind, body and thoughts which together work towards negativity. It is not a disease but an illness wherein a person is not able to do normal things. Due to the depressed state of mind, a person can find the daily chores to be very taxing and is unable to do them. In this state of mind, a person is unhappy and suffers emotionally and mentally rather than physically. Depression may be caused due to mental stress or due to high intake of antibiotics. At times, anxiety may also be the cause of depression. For some people, depression can also be because of the monotonous life. One's own effort to fight depression when complemented with some home remedies work very well in curing depression.

Home Remedies for Depression

- One of the simplest and effective home remedy for treating depression is to add rose petals in a glass of boiling water. Add sugar to the drink and have it.

- Mix 1/8 teaspoon of nutmeg powder with 1 tablespoon of freshly extracted amla juice. Consume this mixture thrice a day.
- Licorice tea also works well for depressed minds. Take 1-3 cups of tea per day to get rid of depression.
- The plant, Griffonia simplicifolia, gives a substance 5HTP which is extracted from the seedpods of the plant. Intake of this would relieve a person from depression.
- Another remedy for curing depression is to have an apple with milk and honey.
- This might surprise you but a neutral immersion bath for about an hour would do wonders in curing a person off depression and uplift his/her mood.
- Dry the root of asparagus and make a powder of it. Daily one or two grams of intake of this powder would heal a person's mind from depression.
- Make a tea and add 1/4-teaspoon basil and 1/2 teaspoon of sage per cup of hot water. Consuming this mixture two times a day would be helpful in relieving a person from depression.
- Boil a cup of hot water. Add powdered seeds of 2 green cardamoms and sugar. Drink this when warm. It would help in treating depression.
- Diet is also an important concern for treating depression. Having a well balanced nutritional food is very essential. Eat a lot of nuts, cheese, apple cider vinegar in a glass of water, pumpkin seeds, carrot juice, apple juice, 5-6 plums, ruta leaves mixed with cumin.
- In 1 cup of rice milk or soy milk, cook 3-4 tablespoons of oatmeal. Add nuts, almonds, dried fruits, maple syrup or honey to it. this would be effective in curing depression.

- Another method would be to stir a tsp of lavender leaves in a cup of boiling water. Have it when warm 3 times a day.
- Yet another natural way to cure depressed mind is to soak feet in a tub with hot water with rosemary leaves, chlorine and some soap added to it. Do this for about 20 minutes and then rub your feet.

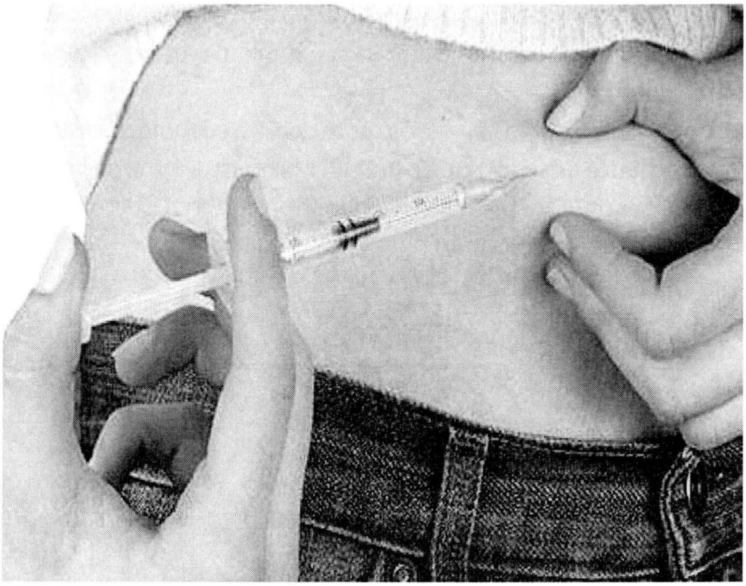

27. Diabetes

Diabetes is a condition when the body has high level of blood glucose and the excretion of the excess glucose in the urine. It is a chronic nutritional disorder. In this case, the body is unable to break the sugar levels and also cannot produce insulin. While the former causes excess of sugar level in the blood, the latter is concerned loss of energy. Diabetes is gradually emerging out as a big problem in the world at large. While the disorder mostly strikes the obese people in middle or older age, it is also common in the youth as well. The normal sugar content should be is 80 -120mg per 100 ml of blood. When it is above this level, it needs to be controlled. Diabetes causes hunger, weight loss, thirst, urination, dehydration. In severe cases also, heart disease, hearing and vision problems are also caused. However, the level of sugar can be controlled with minimum efforts.

Home Remedy for Diabetes

- Having fenugreek seeds water is one of the most effective remedy for treating diabetes. Saturate 90 -100 seeds in

250 liters of water. Keep them overnight. In the morning mash the seeds and strain them. Drink this water everyday.

- Bittermelon or bitter gourd is also beneficial in curing diabetes. A person suffering from diabetes can have half cup juice regularly. Another method would be to fry the bittermelon and add salt and other condiments.
- Take some honey and combine equal amounts of turmeric powder and dried gooseberry powder to it. Have this mixture regularly. Another method would be to mix equal amounts of gooseberry juice and fresh turmeric juice. Intake this mixed juice on an empty stomach daily.
- Mango leaves also fight diabetes. Take about 3-4 mango tree leaves and boil them in water. Have this water when warm.
- For people who have higher sugar level, chew 3-4 leaves of jamun (Syszygium cumini) in the morning and evening. One can also mash 3-4 leaves of jamun tree in half cup of water and drink it.
- Dip 60 grams of fresh ripe fruit in 300 ml of boiling water and cover it. After about half an hour, mash the jamun and strain it. Drink this juice three times a day.
- Mix 3 tablespoons of cinnamon powder to a liter of water. Heat this water for 20 minutes. Strain this mixture and have the water when warm.
- Another easy yet useful home remedy to reduce blood sugar level would be to chew two leaves, each of neem and bilva in the morning.
- Soak a few almonds and keep them overnight. Have them first thing in the morning in an empty stomach.
- Consume ten leaves each of basil, neem and belpatras with a glass of water on an empty stomach in the morning. This would be very useful in treating diabetes.
- Take a jar of water and immerse the peels of green plantain, after it has been washed. Intake this water three to four times in a day.

- Consume 2 tablespoons of apple cider vinegar thrice a day to relieve of diabetes.
- Diabetic patients should increase the consumption of soybeans, celery, cucumbers, string beans, onion and garlic in their diet.

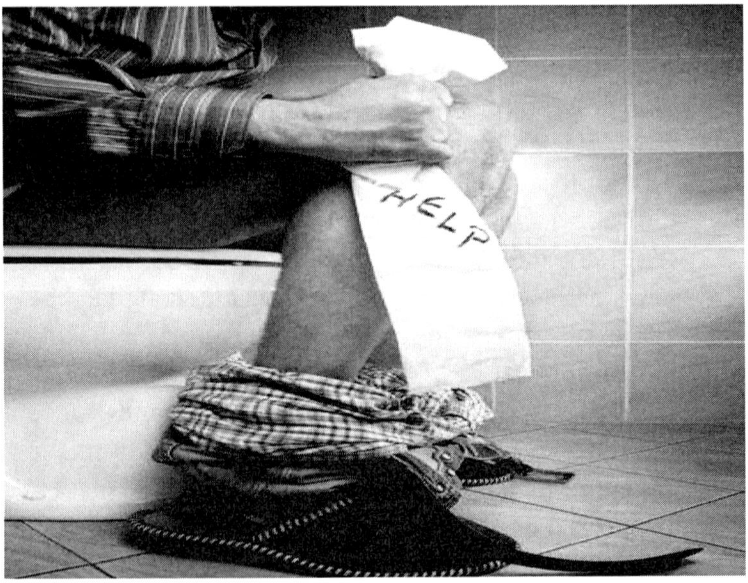

28. Diarrhea

Commonly known as loose motions, diarrhea is the frequent passage of unformed watery loose stools. Diarrhea can be a mild one, acute or chronic. People of any age can be struck with diarrhea. It is a condition where the water is either not absorbed properly or there is excess of water secreted by the organs. The most common symptoms for diarrhea are loose stools, vomiting, stomach pain, thirst, fever, nausea and dehydration. If diarrhea occurs for longer period it can result in general weakness due to loss of various vitamins from the body. Overeating, incomplete digestion of the food, viral or bacterial infection, bowel disorder, food allergies are some of the causes for diarrhea. The most effective way to get rid of diarrhea would be to refer to the natural ways.

Home Remedy for Diarrhea

- A simple and effective remedy for treating diarrhea would be to take banana along with curd.

- Take ½ tsp lemon juice, ½ tsp ginger juice and 1/4 tsp pepper powder. Intake this mixture twice a day.
- Boil to 2 cups of water and allow it to get warm. Mix 3 tsp of black pepper and 1 ½ tsp of kelp to it. Drink this mixture to cure diarrhea.
- Ginger is also effective in treating diarrhea. Intake ginger tea to stop the cramps and pain.
- Drinking lots of fluids would be beneficial in curing diarrhea. . Drinks like ginger ale or carrot juice is good for making the stools less watery. Avoid taking caffeine and alcohol.
- Cook brown rice in water for about 45 minutes. Once cooked, strain the mixture. Have the rice and drink the water in which the rice has been cooked.
- In half cup of boiling water, mix 1 tsp of ginger juice. Drink this mixture when hot after every hour.
- Prepare a paste of lemon along with seeds and add a pinch of salt to it. A tsp of this paste 2-3 times in a day.
- Take 1 tsp of apple cider vinegar in a glass of water with each meal. This is an effective way to cure diarrhea.
- Intake of mango nut powder with water cures diarrhea.
- Take 1/2 tsp of fenugreek seeds and add 1/2 tsp of roasted cumin seeds. Add 4 tsp of yogurt (curd) to it. Have this mixture three times a day.
- Add 4 tablespoons of honey to 8 ounces of water. Have this mixture as it is helpful in treating diarrhea.
- Take fennel and white cumin seeds in equal amounts. Roast this mixture and take this in a dose of 3 grams with water. Have this in a span of three hours.
- Take 200 grams of buttermilk with roasted cumin seeds and half gram of black salt. Drink this mixture to treat diarrhea.
- Drinking starchy liquids such as arrowroot water, barley water, rice gruel and coconut water are highly beneficial in treating diarrhea.

- Take a glass of milk and boil it for 10 minutes. Discard the skin that forms on the milk. Add hot chocolate and drink this.
- Take a cup of cold milk and blend handful of chopped red radishes and ½ tsp of cornstarch. It is a natural way to treat diarrhea.
- Powder 10 grams of dry fruit of Indian gooseberry and 5 grams of black Chebulic myrobalan. Have 1 gram of this mixture two times a day.

29. Discoloration of Lips

Discoloration of the lips is a condition when the color of the lips changes from the usual red or pink to dark shades. It can affect both men and women and is not bounded by age either. Some of the causes of discoloration of lips include smoking, chewing of tobacco, chemotherapy, excessive fluoride use or use of low grade cosmetics. At times, discoloration of the lips can also be a heredity problem. If it is so, the ailment cannot be cured completely. However, retreating to some natural remedies, it can be lightened or treated partially.

Home Remedy for Discoloration of Lips

- The most simple and effective way to cure discoloration of the lip would be to have at least 10 glasses of water per day.
- Lime is a very good bleaching agent. Apply lime juice on the lips every might before bed. This would help in treating discoloration of the lips.
- Sun rays also causes discoloration of the lips. Applying some sunscreen lotion on your lips would help solve this ailment.
- Apply a small amount of clarified butter little every night to soothe lips. Not only, would it cure the discoloration but also help to keep the lips moisturized.
- For people who are in the habit of smoking or in taking caffeinated drinks the first step would be reduce or lessen the intake. This would help in both prevention and treatment of discoloration of lips.
- Make a paste of fresh milk cream in which saffron has been soaked overnight. Apply this paste to cure discoloration of the lips.

30. Dry Chapped Lips

Chapped, dry or cracked lips are a common problem. Unlike the other parts of the skin, lips do not produce natural oils needed to protect against cold winds and low humidity. As such, the lips get dry, cracked or chapped. Some of the symptoms for dry or chapped lips are bleeding, lips that look dried, red and rough, loss of moisture from the lips, slight pain, sensitivity of lips, frequent licking of the lips and tenderness of lips. Over exposure to the sun or cold and windy conditions, infections, allergies to cosmetic products, drugs, dehydration, frequent use of chemicals or soaps are some of the causes for the dryness to occur. However, this can be solved by retreating to the natural ways.

Home Remedy for Dry Chapped Lips

- The most simple and vital treatment for curing dry chapped lips would be intake lots of water. Less water results in dryness in both the skin and the lips. Keeping the body hydrated is very important.
- Another simple yet effective home remedy would be to apply lip balm or petroleum jelly on the lips. This will help them remain smooth. Do not forget to apply it before going to bed.
- Pure ghee or butter is also beneficial in treating dry chapped lips. Apply a little ghee or butter into the naval. It helps to keep the lips smooth and heals the cracks formed.
- Take a few rose petals and soak them in raw milk for a few hours. After this, make a paste and apply it on the

lips. This would not only heal the dryness but also work effectively in retaining the lost pink color.

- Apply milk cream on the lips. This will help remove the dry dead skin and to make the lips smooth.
- Rub a slice of cucumber on your lips. This would help cure dry and chapped lips.
- Grind a few neem leaves and take out the juice. Apply this juice on the lips to heal the cracked and chapped lips.
- Application of aloe vera gel on the lips also cures a person suffering from dry chapped lips.
- Loss of vitamin A is the cause for dry chapped lips. Increase in the intake of foods rich in vitamin A such as carrots, green leafy vegetables and tomatoes, legumes, whole grains and nutritional yeast.
- In a tsp of glycerin, add a few drops of honey. Apply this paste on the lips and keep them overnight. This will help to keep the lips soft and smooth.
- Apply castor oil on the lips. This will help to cure the dry chapped lips.
- Another effective way to cure dry chapped lips would be to apply sun screen lip balm or moisturizer. This would help prevent dry patches and also heal the dryness of the lips.
- For women who put on lipstick, apply moisturizer-based lipstick on the lips. Do not put on excessive lipstick and allow the lips to breathe.
- Crush a few rose petals in glycerin. This would not only retain the color and the lost moister but also cure dryness.
- Avoid wetting the lips with the tongue. It makes the lips dark, and color and lose the moister. Instead apply a chap stick or moisturizer.

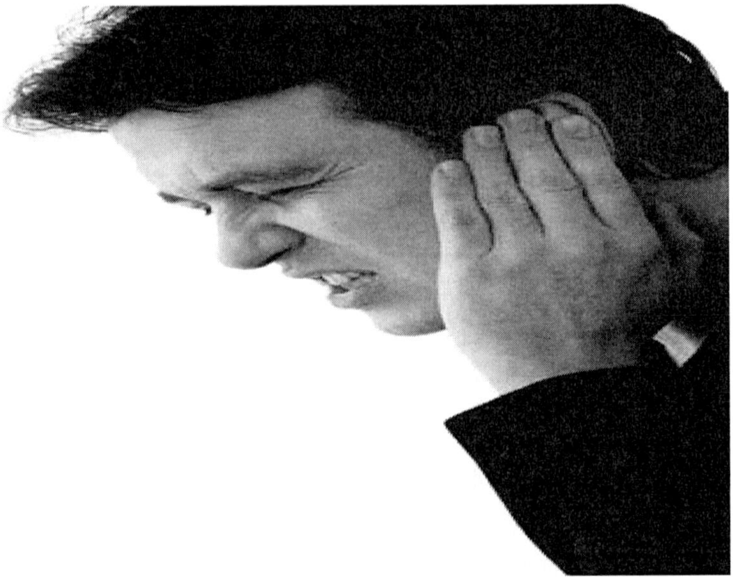

31. Earache

Earache is a common ailment found in children rather than adults. In this particular condition, the Eustachian tubes get plugged. It is a troublesome condition and occurs more in the nighttime. This is because a person stops using the throat muscle. As such, the Eustachian tubes get congested and hence there is more feeling of pain. Some causes for earache are exposure to constant loud sounds, common cold, pressure differences, ear-nose-throat problems, etc. Earache can range from a slight pain to extreme pain and even result in pus formation. However, this can be treated using the natural remedies.

Home Remedy for Earache

- In a tsp of sesame oil, add half a clove of garlic. Heat this until it becomes warm. Lie on the bed and put 4 drops of it. After 10 minutes, change the side and put the oil in the other ear.

- Warm some licorice in ghee and prepare a paste out of it. Apply this mixture externally over the ear. This would help you relieve of the pain.
- Warm some sesame oil and immerse a few leaves of the castor plant. Dab this oil around the ear.
- Take a piece of guggulu herb (Commiphora wightii) and burn it. Switch off the gas when the herb is half burned. Smoke would emit out of the herb. Let the smoke enter the affected area. It would help lessen the apin.
- Take some oil of ajwain and sesame seeds in the ratio of 1:3. Warm this mixture and apply it in the ear. Four drops of this would be effective in treating earache.
- Immerse four to five cloves of garlic in some linseed oil and burn it. Strain the oil and store it in a bottle. Apply this oil every morning and evening to get relieved from earache.
- Grind some basil leaves to form a paste. Warm this at room temperature. Once it becomes at a bearable temperature, put four to five drops of this oil in the ears.
- Take a few mango leaves and extract the juice. Warm this juice a little and apply it on the ear putting four drops at each ear. This would help cure earache.
- Chop a radish into small pieces. Immerse this into mustard oil and warm it. Store this oil in a glass bottle and put a few drops when there is pain.
- Extract some ginger juice and put a few drops of it in the ear. Warm this and put four drops of it. This would help treat earache.
- Extract the juice of the onion and warm it a little. Put four drops of it in each ear while going to sleep.
- Another effective home remedy would be to put four drops warmed mustard oil into the ears.
- If the earache is due to swimming, put few drops of mineral oil in each ear before going to swim. It is helpful in treating earache.

- If the earache is due to flying, pop in some candy or chewing gum. Work the throat muscle as this would relieve from the earache.
- Add fenugreek seed to mustard or linseed oil. Warm this oil and filter it. Once cooled, put it in each ear in four to five drops.

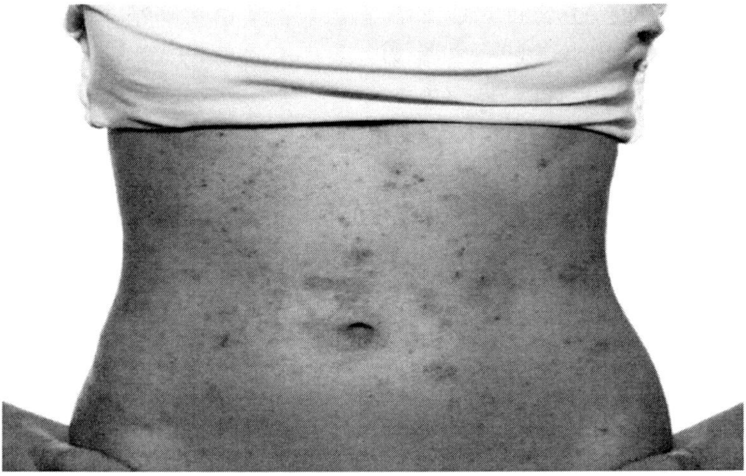

32. Eczema

Eczema is a group of skin disorder which has derived its name from a Greek word which means 'to boil'. A chronic skin disorder, it is the result of inflammation of the skin which results in the formation of eruptions in the skin. Eczema is mostly formed in children and infants and is seldom seen among adults. Also called dermatitis, eczema is a non contagious disease. The various causes of eczema are allergies, varicose veins, cold and dry weather, nutritional deficiencies, etc. Its symptoms include itching, redness, dryness and flakiness of the skin. The most common affected regions are the hands, wrists, arms, neck, face, upper chest and back of the knees. Eczema, however, can be cured naturally.

Home Remedy for Eczema

- A simple way to cure eczema would be to apply coconut oil on the affected region. This is would help to keep the skin smooth and soft.
- Mudpack when applied in the affected area is also helpful in treating eczema.
- In a tsp of sandalwood paste, add a tsp of camphor. Apply this paste on the eczema affected area. This is helpful in curing eczema.

- Another effective remedy would be making a paste using 1 tablespoon each of turmeric powder and bitter neem leaves. Apply this paste to the affected areas.
- Eczema can also be treated using water. Cold compress or cold wet fomentations when applied two times a day is found beneficial in treating eczema.
- Take some almond leaves and mash them in water. Apply this mashed mixture on the eczema affected region. It would be helpful in curing eczema.
- An effective natural remedy for treating eczema would be to rub nutmeg against a smooth stone with a few drops of water. A paste would be formed. Application of this is a useful way to cure eczema.
- Take an iron vessel and boil 200 grams of mustard oil in it. Add 50 grams of fresh clean leaves of neem in it. Once the leaves turn black, let it cool and then strain it. Apply this oil 4 times a day to cure eczema.
- Mashed papaya seeds when applied on the eczema affected area reduce itching and help a person suffering from eczema.
- Dab some witch hazel on the affected area with a cotton ball. Apply this on the affected area.
- Application of spearmint leaf juice also helps reduce eczema.
- Sun bathing is also helpful in curing eczema. It kills the harmful bacteria and thus treating the inflammation caused.
- It is generally advisable to avoid using soaps, chemicals and other drying agents on the eczema affected area.
- Mix 1 tsp. comfrey root, 1 tsp. white oak bark, 1 tsp. slippery elm bark in 2 cups of water. Let this mixture boil for about 35 minutes. Wash the eczema affected area with this.

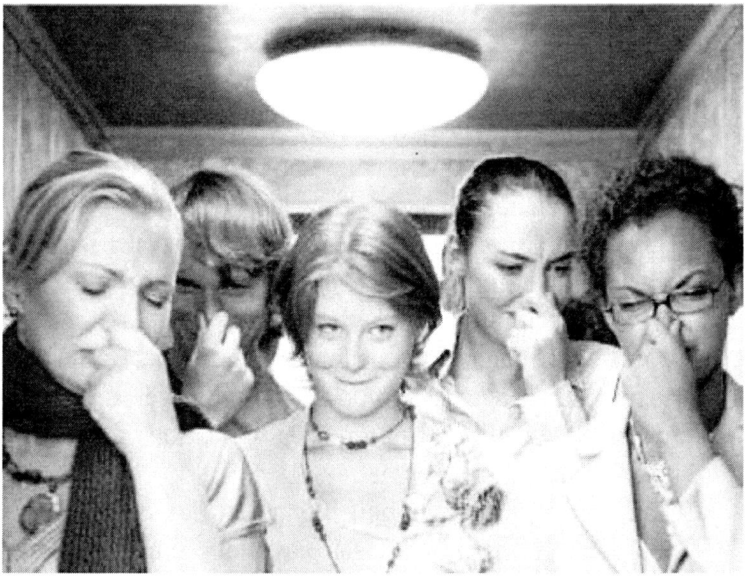

33. Flatulence

Flatulence is the emission of gases present in the intestine. The mixture of gases 'flatus' is released under pressure and creates a sound accompanied by a foul odor. Apart from causing discomfort and pain due to bloating, it also causes social embarrassment. The most common symptoms of flatulence or more popularly known as gas are a feeling of bloating and discomfort, excessive expulsion of wind, belching and pain in the abdomen. The problem of flatulence is very common and usually due to dietary reasons. Problems in digesting certain types of food cause flatulence. While for some it might be due to lactose intolerance, the others may suffer it because of grain based food. Yet, others might suffer due to foods which are heavy in carbohydrates. Flatulence, however, is not a serious problem and can be cured using natural treatments.

Home Remedy for Flatulence

- Do not forget the basics of eating as this is the most natural and effective way to treat flatulence. Eat slowly and chew the food thoroughly. Do not gulp the food. This is the best way to cure the problem of gas.

- In a cup of warm water, add 1/2 tsp of dry ginger powder with a pinch each of asafetida and rock salt. Drink this mix to get relieved from gas.
- Take a cup of lukewarm water and add 2 tsp of brandy. Intake this before going to bed.
- Soak some ginger slices in lemon juice. Chew this after every meal. This would help cure gas.
- In a tsp of honey, add a drop of dill oil. Intake this after every meal to help treat flatulence.
- Grind 1 tsp of pepper, 1 tsp of dry ginger and 1 tsp of green cardamom seeds. Add ½ tsp of this mixture in water and drink it one hour after meal.
- Peppermint also proves effective in treating flatulence. Not only does it refreshes the breath, but also cures gas.
- Peppermint tea is also effective in treating flatulence. The other tea includes anise tea, spearmint tea, and caraway tea. Spearmint or peppermint candy would also do the trick.
- Avoid foods such as beans, cabbage, cauliflower, broccoli, yeast-containing foods such as breads and cheese. Carbonated drinks also produce gas.
- Do not drink water after 15 minutes or during meals. It weakens the digestive system.

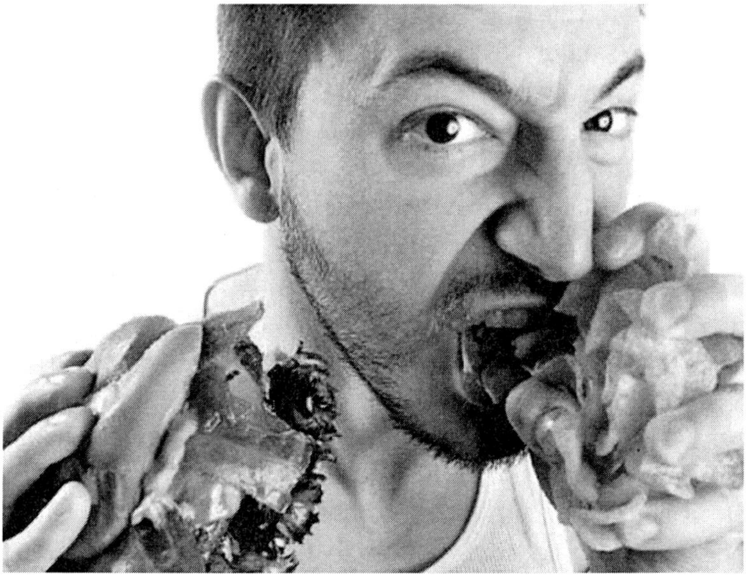

34. Gaining Weight

The problem of being underweight has become a common phenomenon. It is a condition, when a person does not have an ideal weight, according to his/her height and sex. A person, who weighs almost 10 to 20 percent below the average, is termed underweight. Some of the causes for underweight problems are rise in the stress level, lack of sleep, poor nutrition, exposure to pollutants, lack of exercise, etc. Bad eating habits also add to the causes for the occurrence of the problem. Being underweight can also arise due to hereditary reasons. Apart from being skinny, a person starts facing a number of health problems. However, gaining weight is not as major problem and can be treated by indulging in the right kind of eating habit.

Home Remedy for Gaining Weight

- The most effective and simple remedy to gain weight is to consume banana milk shake. It is a fast way to gain weight.

- Another effective way would be to have banana thrice a day. This should be followed with curd or milk.
- Muskmelon is beneficial in treating underweight problem. Have muskmelon three times a day as it helps in gaining weight.
- Another effective way to cure underweight problem would be to have fruit diet with milk. While fruits nourish the body with sugar, milk provides the proteins.
- An effective way to gain weight would be consume a glass of hot milk with a tablespoon of honey.
- Take a cup of milk and put some almonds, date palm and anjeer in it. Boil this milk and have it when warm. This is helpful in treating underweight problem.
- Mangoes are useful in gaining weight. Have a mango followed by a glass of milk. The other way would be to have a glass of mango milk shake every day for a month.
- Raisins are beneficial in solving underweight problems. Have 30 grams of raisins every day for about a month. This would surely cure underweight problems.
- Take 3-4 dry figs and immerse them in water. Keep them overnight. Have this twice a day to get cured of underweight problem.
- Combine equal amounts of pomegranate seed powder, white muesli powder and Indian ginseng root powder. Intake this mixture, twice a day for about a month, along with a glass of water or milk. Not only does it helps gain weight, but also tones up the body. Intake 100 to 150 grams of bran with fruits. The best deal would be to take it with papaya. It works as an excellent appetizer improving digestion and reducing constipation.
- Increase in the intake of fatty foods such as flour, rice honey, raisins, figs, dates, butter, germinated wheat, etc.

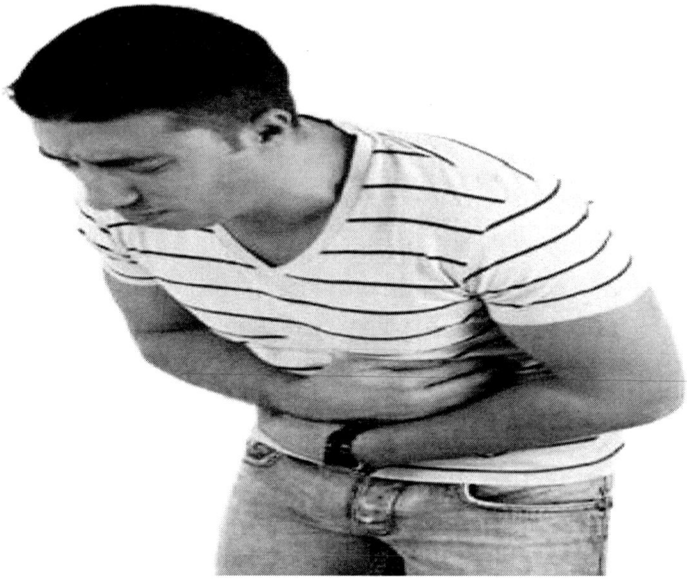

35. Gastritis

A swelling or an inflammation caused in the mucus membrane lining of the stomach is called gastritis. Gastritis can either be a mild or acute. In some cases, it can also be chronic or severe. The most common symptoms for gastritis are loss of appetite, nausea, vomiting, headache and dizziness. It also causes pain and discomfort in the stomach. The other symptoms include coated tongue, foul breath, bad taste in the mouth, increased flow of saliva, scanty urination, a general feeling of uneasiness, and mental depression. The best way to cure or treat gastritis would be to turn to the natural remedies.

Home Remedy for Gastritis

- One of the simplest and effective home remedy to cure gastritis would be to take a tsp of ajwain with a pinch of salt. Gulp this mixture with a glass of lukewarm water.
- Coconut water also proves to be effective in treating gastritis. Take coconut water twice a day.

- Another good remedy for curing gastritis is to make a combination of 200 ml of spinach juice and 300 ml of carrot juice. Drink this combination once a day.
- Apply heat through hot bags or hot water bottle in an empty stomach. This is effective in curing the problem of gastritis.
- Intake half cup of potato juice before meals. It is a natural way to treat gastritis.
- Take a cup of hot water and put a half a tsp of licorice root tea. Boil the water for about 10 minutes after which strain it. Drink this concoction when warm. Repeat this at least thrice a day.
- Increase in the consumption of water and juices also help to get relieved from gastritis.
- In 125 grams of curd, add 2 grams of Sprague and half gram of black salt. Have this mixture as it is effective in relieving gastritis problem.
- Combine Sprague powder and black salt in the ratio of 6:1. Intake 2 grams of this mixture, along with warm water. This is a good natural remedy to cure gastritis.
- Buttermilk and curd also works well to cure gastritis. Have buttermilk and curd along with asafetida and cumin water.
- Take 2 teaspoons of peach leaves in a cup and add boiling water to it. After about 10 minutes, drink this concoction. Have this mixture thrice a day.
- Take a few figs and immerse it in warm water. After about 10 minutes, strain this water and drink it.
- Chew roasted fennel after meals. This provides relief from gastritis.
- Intake a cup of rice gruel two times a day. This would impart relief from the problem of gastritis.
- Chewing fresh ginger before taking meals is also helpful in preventing and curing gastritis.

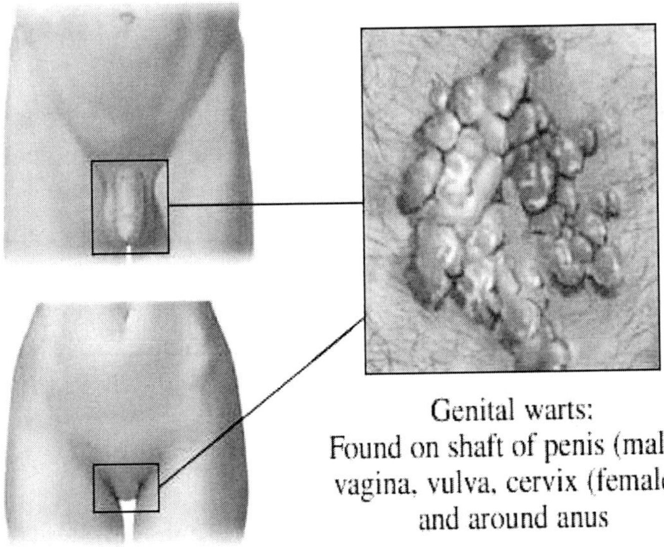

Genital warts:
Found on shaft of penis (male), vagina, vulva, cervix (female), and around anus

36. Genital Warts

Genital warts grow on the penis and in and around the entrance to the vagina and anus. They are caused by a family of viruses known as human papillomavirus (HPV) that are transmitted during sexual intercourse. The CDC estimates that there are 5.5 million new cases of genital warts in the United States each year. Genital warts are treatable with topical medications and can be removed with minor surgical procedures. Certain types of HPV that cause genital infections can also cause cervical cancer. Regular pap smear screenings can detect cervical cancer in an early stage, when the disease is easier to treat.

Genital Warts home remedy treatment is quite effective. Following are some Genital Warts cure home remedies.

Home Remedy for Genital Warts

- Apply oil (vitamin E) on the genital warts affected area and put some chopped raw garlic pieces on it and cover using an adhesive tape.

- Extract juice from onion slices and add salt to it. Apply this juice on the wart-affected area and see the magical effects.
- Another great idea is to apply the milky juice of figs on the warts 2-3 times in a day, till the warts disappear.
- Put few drops of apple cider vinegar on the warts using cotton ball.
- Consume foods rich in folic acid and beta-carotene. Eat plenty of green leafy veggies.

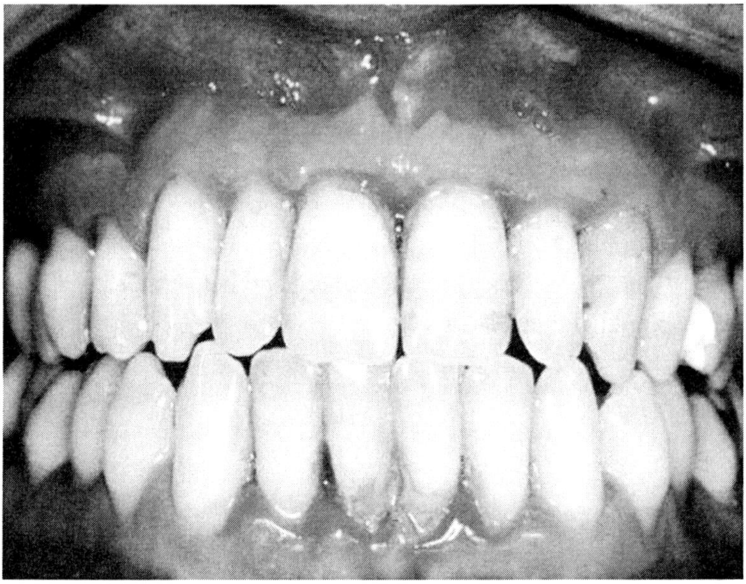

37. Gingivitis

Gingivitis or bleeding gums is an inflammation caused in the mouth. It affects the tissues surrounding teeth and gums. A periodontal disease, gingivitis may turn into serious tooth problems, if not treated on time. It can also lead to the destruction of bone and tooth loss. Gingivitis is caused due to plaque, bacteria and food particles accumulation between the gums and the teeth. Though this might look a menial affair, the accumulation emits toxic elements. These elements, in turn, cause the inflammation of the gums. Some of the symptoms of gingivitis are painful gums, bleeding while brushing, red gums, swollen gums, tender gums, bad breath and bad taste in mouth. However, gingivitis can be treated at home following some natural remedies.

Home Remedy for Gingivitis

- The best home remedy to cure gingivitis would be to brush twice regularly. Use herbal toothpaste and herbal mouthwash.

- One of the most effective natural remedies to cure gingivitis is to rub the gums with clove oil. There may be burning sensation but it would heal the ailment. Another method would be to chew a piece of clove in the mouth.
- Toothpaste containing mint, babool, neem, holy basil would be the best deal to fight gingivitis. Not only do they avoid the spreading of the infection, but also reduce the swelling or inflammation.
- Gargling also helps treat gingivitis. Take a glass of lukewarm water and add a pinch of salt to it. Gargle with this concoction, twice a day.
- Gargling with triphala concoction is beneficial in curing gingivitis. In a glass of lukewarm water, add a tsp of triphala powder. Gargle with this combination.
- Aloe vera proves helpful in treating gingivitis. Rub the aloe vera pulp in the mouth. After rubbing once, gargle with water. Repeat the process a few times.
- Combine 2 tsp of white oak bark herbal powder, 1 tsp of myrrh herbal powder, ¾ tsp of peppermint leaves' powder, 1/8 tsp of clove powder. Grind this mixture and store it in an air tight container. Have 1 tablespoon of this mixture every morning and night. Rub this in the affected area of the mouth.
- Make a mixture of baking soda and water. Dab the affected area with a finger and then brush with the herbal powder. Not only would it heal but also neutralize the acidity of bacteria.
- Take equal amounts of 3% solution of Hydrogen Peroxide and water. Gargle with this combination but make sure that it is not consumed.
- Increase in the consumption of fresh fruits and vegetables. Include foods rich in fiber and vitamin C and those that have low saturated fats.

- Cranberry juice proves worthwhile in treating gingivitis. Intake cranberry juice but make sure that it does not have sugar.
- It is advisable for a person to use mouthwash that contains sage oil, peppermint oil, menthol, chamomile tincture, etc. Toothpaste containing sage oil, peppermint oil would be effective in treating gingivitis.

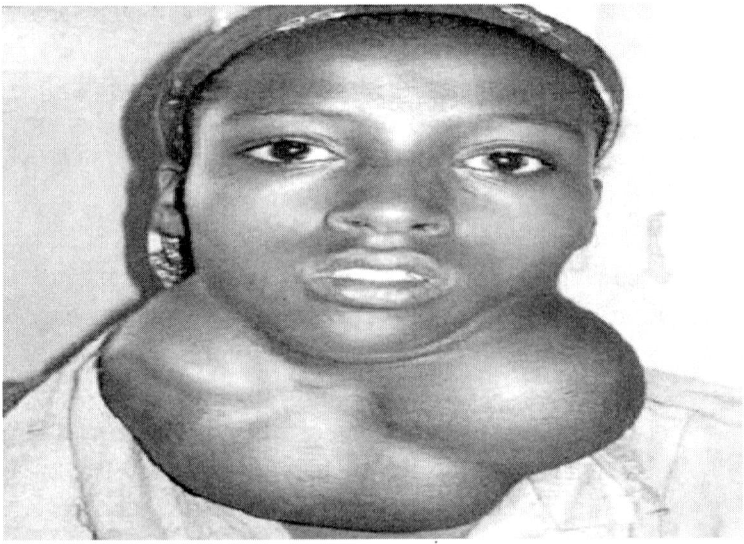

38. Goiter

A disease of the thyroid gland, goiter is a condition which causes swelling at the back of the neck. The size of the swelling ranges from being very small to a visible one. It might turn out to be a very large one. The major causes of goiter are deficiency of iodine in the diet and physical and emotional disturbances. The most common symptom of goiter is the enlargement or swelling of the thyroid gland. Other symptoms include loss of concentration, mood swings, emotionally upset, irritation and even depression. The treatment of the goiter depends on the size and cause of the goiter swelling. Inflamed goiter is painful but if the enlargement is too large, it may also cause difficulty in breathing and swallowing. Goiter can be treated at home.

Home Remedy for Goiter

- A simple remedy to cure goiter would be to use dandelion leaves and ghee. Smear the leaves of dandelion with ghee. Warm it and bandage it over the affected area. Repeat this procedure for about two weeks.

- Ground the seeds of flax in water and heat it. Apply this on the swollen area. Then, bandage the leaves of the tree over it. It is a useful remedy for curing goiter.
- A simple way would be to do the neck stretches and exercises daily. These help stretch the muscles that are attached to the thyroid gland. Aerobics and jogging also help relieve a person suffering from goiter.
- Include barley water in the regular diet. Have it at least once every day to as it proves worthwhile in curing goiter.
- Take 1 tsp of the juice of the leaves of swamp cabbage with tea almonds. Consuming this combination once or twice a day is beneficial in treating goiter.
- A change in diet would be helpful in treating goiter. Include iron rich food in the diet such as guavas, strawberries, citrus fruits, egg yolk, sea food, whole rice, tomatoes, oats, onion, garlic, carrots and lettuce.
- Prepare a decoction of Kachnas (Bauhini variegate). Have 30 ml of decoction of bark two times a day regularly in an empty stomach.
- In case of an infant suffering from goiter, mother's milk is the best home remedy to treat goiter.
- Cool showers every morning and evening proves beneficial in curing the thyroid malfunction.
- Go for four to five smaller meals a day instead of having two to three large meals. This helps digest the food better.
- For people who cannot avoid rice form their diet, consume the old variety of rice instead of the new one.
- Watercress a very good source of iodine. Make a paste of it and apply on the affected area. This would help reduce the swelling. The other method would be to take 2 tablespoon of watercress juice diluted in water thrice for six weeks.

- Regularly intake of water nut (shingara) lotus reed, stem to the lotus tube of Plancuperous tuberosus and pineapple. This would help treat goiter.
- Take equal parts of sorrel leaves and olive oil and mash them. Spread this paste on the goiter. It would help relieve a person suffering from goiter.

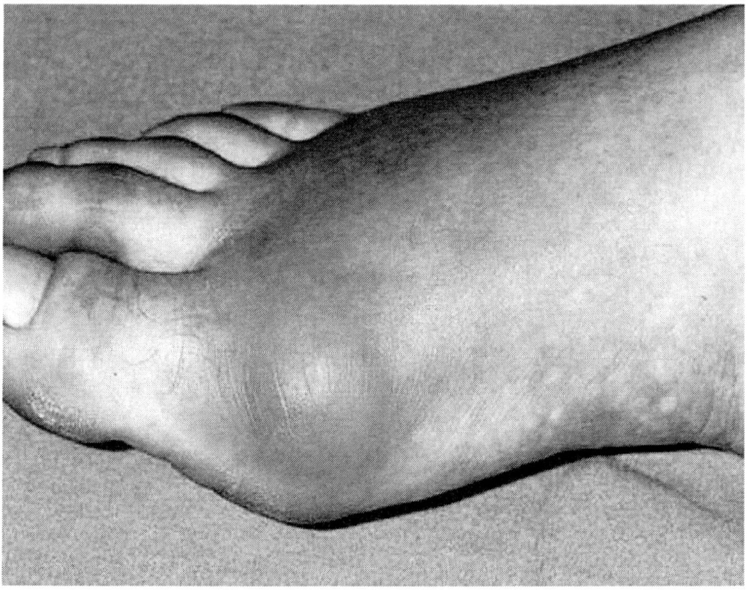

39. Gout

Gout is a condition when there is excess of uric acid deposits in the body. It is a type of arthritis. In this case, the minimum level of uric acid present in the body increases. As such, these deposit in the joints, instead of being flushed into the kidneys. Gout mainly causes swollenness or inflammation which is usually seen in the knees, feet, hands, wrists and elbows. At times, deposition is also seen in the areas below the skin and in the kidneys and the urinary tract. It is noted that the symptoms of gout are usually visible only in the night. The most common symptoms are pain and inflammation in the joints, swelling and feeling of pressure in the area where the swelling has occurred. Unhealthy diet is the prime cause for gout. It can however, be treated using some home remedies.

Home Remedy for Gout

- In a glass of water, squeeze half lemon. Take this concoction three times a day. Since lemon is rich in vitamin C, it helps in dissolving the gouty deposits.

- Intake 6 to 8 ounces of fluid per day. Not only would it lessen the gout attack, but would also prevent kidney stones from developing.
- French beans are helpful in treating gout. Extract half a cup of juice and drink this once or twice everyday. It would provide a healing effect and also reduce inflammation.
- Grind mustard powder and mix equal proportion of whole wheat powder. Add water to this mixture to make a paste. Apply this paste over the affected area.
- Take 2 tsp each of organic apple cider vinegar and honey. Consume this mixture once a day.
- Take a bucket of warm water and add two cups of Epsom salt in it. Dip the feet in it until the water loses its heat.
- Dip a white flannel cloth in warm castor oil. Place this over the affected area. Cover it with a plastic and apply heating pads to it.
- For temporary relief, apply ice cubes over the affected area. This would reduce the pain instantly.
- Combine one cup each of vinegar and water. Add 1tsp of pepper to it. Dab this mixture on the painful joint and keep it for about 2 to 3 hours.
- Consume 3-4 bananas everyday. Since bananas are rich in minerals like phosphorus, it would react with the uric deposits thus eliminating them.
- For people who suffer from gout in their toes, fill the bathtub with water and add one-third cup of ground ginger in it. Soak the affected area for about 30 minutes, after which, rinse thoroughly.
- Regularly exercising works well to treat gout problem. The exercise should focus on the joints. Stretching joints and muscles would help to maintain a range of motion.

- Increase in the consumption of foods rich in vitamin C such as citrus fruits, berries, tomatoes, green pepper and leafy green vegetables.
- Apples, cherries and strawberries are beneficial in treating gout.

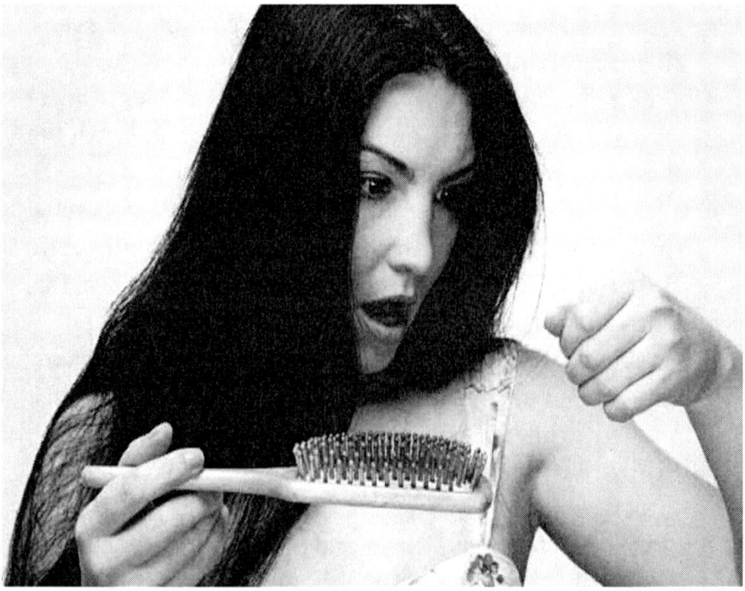

40. Hair Loss

Hair loss is a condition when a person faces extreme hair fall. Baldness as it is referred to, can be due to hereditary reasons, medication or even because of medical conditions. A little bit of hair fall every day is normal and is part of the growth cycle but when the hair loss becomes a little more than the usual, it might cause baldness. This can affect all - men, women and children. The major factor for hair loss is nutritional deficiency. Other causes are age factor, genetic factor, hormonal changes, stress and excessive dandruff. Hair loss must be treated on time as the risk for getting bald increases every time you have a major hair fall. Baldness can be treated at home using some natural remedies.

Home Remedy for Hair Loss

- Take a pot of water and soak few fenugreek seeds in it. Massage it in the scalp and wrap a cloth for about 3 hours. Repeat this procedure for a month to get treated of hair loss.

- Take uncooked egg yolk and massage it on the scalp. Keep it for an hour and then wash off.
- Red henna is beneficial in treating hair loss problem. Smear henna over the scalp and keep it for an hour. Wash the hair. Repeat this process in a span of 10 to 15 days.
- Apply castor oil on the scalp and the roots but not on the hair. Wrap the hair with newspaper and tie it with cloth. Keep it overnight and wash it in the morning. Repeat this for 7 to 10 days.
- In a cup of boiling water, add a tsp of mustard seeds. Cook it for about 5 minutes and allow it to cool. Once cooled, drink this concoction.
- Rub olive oil in the scalp. This would help reduce hair loss.
- Take a few rosemary leaves and boil them in water. Strain the combination and store the liquid. Use this concoction daily to rinse the hair with.
- Combine 2 tablespoons of olive oil, rosemary, 1 lemon juice and 1 egg yolk. Apply this mixture on the hair roots and keep it for half an hour. Then, wash off this mixture.
- Extract juice from green coriander leaves. Apply this juice on the head. This proves worthwhile in treating hair loss.
- Boil water and put blanch scented geranium leaves in it. Strain the water and allow it to cool. When cool, wash the hair with it.
- In ½ cup olive oil, add 1 tablespoon of cumin. Rub this over the scalp and leave it for half an hour. Rinse the hair later.
- Grind myrtle leaves and soak it in water for a day. Apply this combination the next night before going to sleep and wrap it with a cloth. Keep it overnight. Wash the hair the next morning with cold or warm water. repeat this procedure for 2 weeks.

- In a ½ cup of coconut oil, add some dry pieces of amla. Boil this mixture and when cool apply it on the scalp. This is beneficial in reducing hair loss.
- Applying coconut milk is also beneficial in treating hair loss. Massage the hair roots with this and rinse it after some time.

41. Halitosis

Halitosis, or more popularly known as bad breath, is a condition when an unpleasant odor emits out from the oral cavity of a person. It has become a very common ailment. The origin of the bad breath is mainly from the mouth but at times non oral parts such as upper and lower respiratory tracts, the gastrointestinal tract, and some diseases involving the kidneys may also be the reason. The major causes for halitosis are Poor dental hygiene, tooth infections, smoking, diabetes, hiatus hernia, etc. The remnants of food deposits settling in the tongue or mouth also give scope for the growth and breeding of bacteria. Apart from being destructive for the mouth, it is also a social embarrassment and needs to be treated.

Home Remedy for Halitosis

- The simplest and the most effective home remedy to cure halitosis would be to take fenugreek tea. Make a tea using fenugreek seeds. Intake this tea regularly.
- Chewing raw green guava is helpful in curing bad breath. It would serve very helpful in treating halitosis.
- In 2 cups of water, add several sprigs of coarsely chopped parsley so that it steeps in water. Add 2 to 3 whole cloves or a tsp of powdered cloves. Strain this mixture and use it as a mouth wash.
- Cardamoms can be used as a mouth freshner and helps in treating halitosis. Chew cardamom after meals and in between the long intervals. This would surely cure a person from bad breath.
- Deep breaths are helpful in curing halitosis. Perform pranayam at least half an hour every day.

- Include a lot of vegetables and fruits in the regular diet. This would act beneficially in solving the problem of halitosis.
- Rinsing the mouth with baking soda helps in solving the problem of halitosis. Mix baking soda in a cup of water. Gargle with this water.
- Squeeze a lemon and add a little honey to it. Have this mixture two times a day both, in the morning and evening. This would be useful in treating bad breath problem.
- Add 2 to 3 drops of oil of oregano in the drinking water. this would help solve the problem of halitosis.
- Chewing mint leaves is also beneficial in curing a person who is suffering from bad breath or halitosis.
- Choose a mouth wash which contains eucalyptol and thymol. Derived from eucalyptus and thyme respectively, these proved worthwhile in destroying bad breath.
- Increase in the intake of foods rich in vitamins C and E. These help in reducing the bad breath.
- It is advisable that people suffering from bad breath should brush their teeth immediately after consuming food rich in sulfur.
- It is very important to have a well balanced diet. Have foods that consist of seeds, nuts, vegetables, grains and fruits.

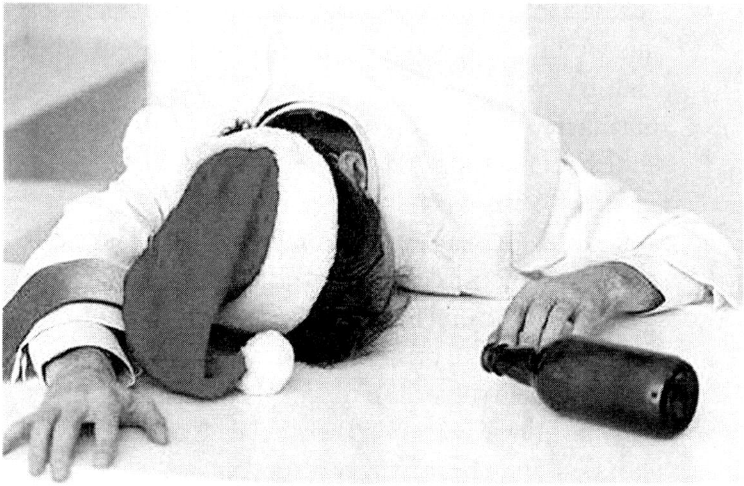

42. Hangover

Hangover can be termed as one of the after effects of consuming alcohol. It is almost experienced by 3/4th of the drinkers. People who take in alcohol experience a hangover at one or the other point. There are various causes of hangover ranging from drinking much in less time, drinking with an empty stomach, lack of sleep, dehydrated body and poor health. The most common symptoms found during hangover are an upset stomach, a headache, a bad taste in mouth and a guilty conscience. It is not a condition to get tensed about as retreating to some home remedies can cure hangover in a short span of time.

Home Remedies for Hangover

- The best remedy to cure hangover at home would be to increase the intake of vitamin C in the body. Consume fresh citrus fruit juice in large amounts in the morning to cure hangover.
- Another simple remedy which is effective would be to increase in the intake of water. Higher levels of water counter effects the alcohol levels in the body thus curing hangover.

- Lime juice is also beneficial in treating hangover. Take a glass of water and add lime to it. Drink this solution.
- Have several cups of strong coffee. This would reduce or lessen the effect. Tomato juice, peppermint tea or ginger tea also proves worthwhile in treating hangover.
- Consuming a tablespoon of honey would also be beneficial in treating a person who's on a high with alcohol. Since honey has higher levels of fructose, it would act favorably.
- Take a bowl of cold/ chilled water. Dip a handkerchief and apply it on the forehead. This would provide instant relief from the headache caused and also lessen the hangover.
- In 8 ounces of water, add 2 tsp of fresh lime juice and a tsp of sugar. Drink this mixture slowly sip by sip. It would relieve a aperson from the hangover.
- Taking hot water bath the next morning will also be helpful in treating a person who has had alcohol the previous night. It would drain away all the toxins.
- Peel the banana and immerse the peels in a cup of water. Cool this water and drink it. This would helpful in treating in hangover.
- A good cure to relieve a person from hangover would be to make him/her drink chocolate milk before going to bed.
- Make a cup of black coffee without sugar. Add a few drops of lemon juice to it. Drink this concoction. This is an effective remedy to treat hangovers.
- Take a cup of hot water and immerse 5 to 6 crushed thyme leaves in it. Simmer it for about 5 minutes and then strain the tea. When warm, drink this tea. It would provide relief from hangover.
- Having food during and after drinking would help in reducing the effect of hangover.

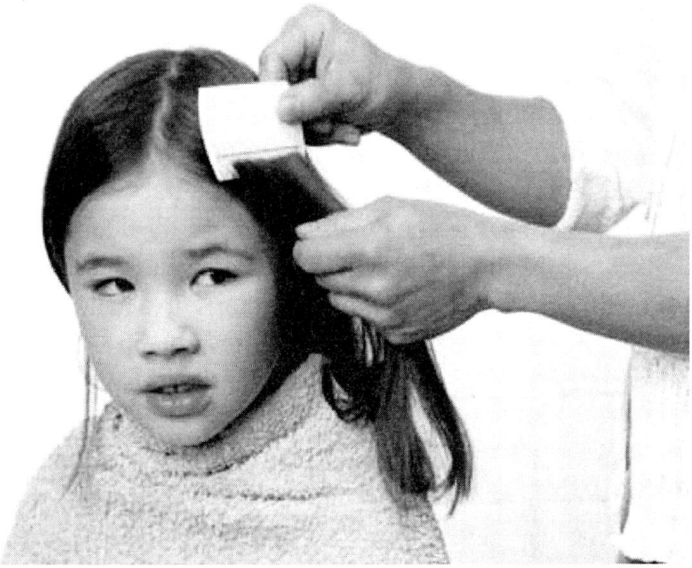

43. Head Louse

Head louse is the presence of ectoparasites on the human hair. While it is more often seen in children, adults are not spared from it completely. For some people, it occurs during some seasons of the year, while the rest have them at anytime. The presence of lice weakens the roots of the hair and also causes hair fall. Apart from being unhygienic, these are also social embarrassment for the person suffering. Lice may be caused due to untidy hair, improper maintenance of long hair, staying with a person who is already suffering from it or using chemical-based shampoo, etc. once infected, lice should be removed instantly and the best way to do it would be to adhere to the natural ways. In the following lines, we provide the home remedies to treat/ cure head louse.

Home Remedy for Head Louse

- One of the effective remedy for treating head louse would be to extract the juice from an onion. Apply this juice on the scalp of the head and keep it for 3 to 4 hours.

Thereafter, shampoo the hair. Repeat this process for 3 days.

- Grind a raw custard apple with its seeds. Store the powder in an air tight box and apply it on the scalp before going to bed. Tie a cloth bandage on it. Have a head wash the next morning.
- Alternatively, custard apple powder can be used to make a paste using some water. Apply this paste and keep it overnight. Wash the hair the next morning. Not only would it clear the lice and the nits, but also keep the dandruff away.
- Mix 6 tsp of water and 2 tsp of vinegar. Dab this mixture on the scalp and tie a cloth bandage over it. Keep it overnight. Apply this mixture two times a week.
- Oil the hair using tea tree oil or any other essential oil at the night. Have a head wash the next morning.
- Another way to use the tea tree oil would be to add 10-15 drops of it into the shampoo. Use this shampoo as a hair wash.
- Oil the hair using mayonnaise oil. Keep it for two hours. Thereafter, comb the hair.
- Take 3 to 4 tsp of butter and add a few drops of lemon to it. Apply this mixture on the head and keep it for some time. (20 seconds given) Wash the hair thoroughly.
- Combine equal quantity of baby oil and vinegar. Apply this combination on the scalp and keep it for an hour. Later, rinse thoroughly using a shampoo.
- Have a head wash and then apply Listerine. Keep it for about 10 to 15 minutes after which, rinse the hair using water.
- Make a paste using 8 to 10 almonds. In this, add 2 to 3 tsp of lime juice. Apply this paste and leave it for ½ an hour. Rinse the hair thoroughly.

- Take 1 tsp each of garlic and lime juice and make a paste. Apply this paste and keep it for half an hour. Thereafter, have a head wash.
- Take an apple and chop it into small pieces. Apply these pieces into the hair. Massage it well for about half an hour. Later, wash the hair. Repeat this for three days.
- Add some camphor to a freshly extracted coconut oil. Keep this overnight. Wash the hair the next morning. Repeat this process for at least 4 days.

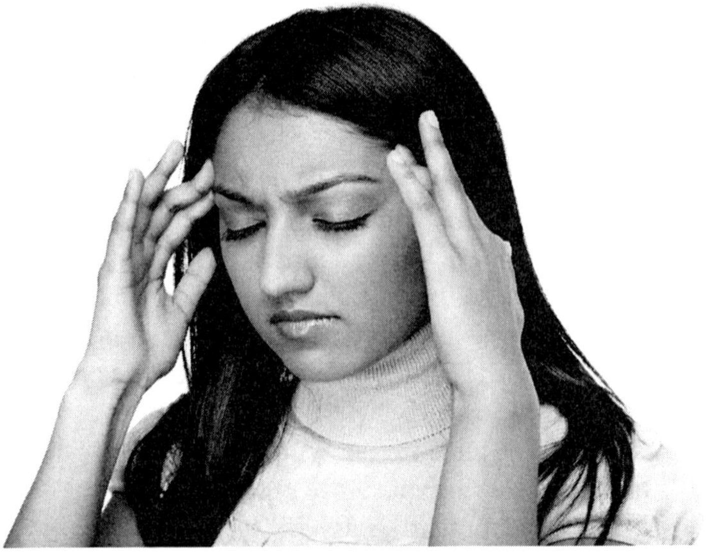

44. Headache

Headache is a common ailment found in the society today. Almost everyone suffers from it at one point or the other. Generally, tension headaches are found in people. This occurs when prolonged tension produces a contraction of the muscles in the back of the neck. The other kinds of headache are migraine and cluster headache. While the former is the hereditary condition and occurs due to inheritance, the latter is the recurring types and occurs for days and months at a stretch. The most common symptoms of headache are aches and tightness around head, behind the eyes, and neck, depression or excitation and blurring of visions. There are number of causes due to which headache is caused. Some of them are allergy, emotional stress and tension, eye strain, high blood pressure or low blood sugar, exposure to extreme temperatures, etc. headaches may be mild or chronic. These, however, can be treated at home using some natural remedies/ home remedies.

Home Remedy for Headache

- A simple yet effective remedy for headache would be to apply a sandalwood powder paste over the forehead. Let the paste dry. Once dry, rub it and then wash.
- Grind a few watermelon seeds and Cuseus grass separately. Mix the grinded powder in equal amounts. Consume 3 grams of this mixture two times a day.
- Take some ginger powder and moisten it. Apply this over the forehead. It is beneficial in treating headache.
- For people who have chronic headache, drinking a glass of water mixed with a tsp of honey in an empty stomach is the best way to deal with it.
- Watermelon juice mixed with sugar works well for headaches due to exposure to excessive heat.
- Mix ½ tsp of mustard seeds powder and in 3 tsp of water. Put this in the nostrils to cure headache and migraine.
- Massage the forehead by rosemary oil. This would provide relief from headache.
- For headache caused due to cold, warm water gargling, nasal cleaning with warm water and steam inhalation would be beneficial.
- Make a paste using 3-4 cloves. Apply this paste on the forehead. It would provide instant relief from the headache.
- Put 2 to 4 drops of cow's butter or ghee in the nostrils for about seven days. This is an effective remedy for headache caused due to sinusitis.
- For headaches which are due to liver or stomach problem, hot fomentations over the abdomen region would provide relief.
- Prepare a paste using lemon crust and water. Apply this paste all over the forehead. This would provide relief from the headache.

- If the headache is because of exposure to cold air, make a paste with the help of 1 tsp each of finely ground cinnamon and water. Apply this paste on the forehead.
- Consuming freshly sliced apple each day empty stomach cures all the chronic headaches.

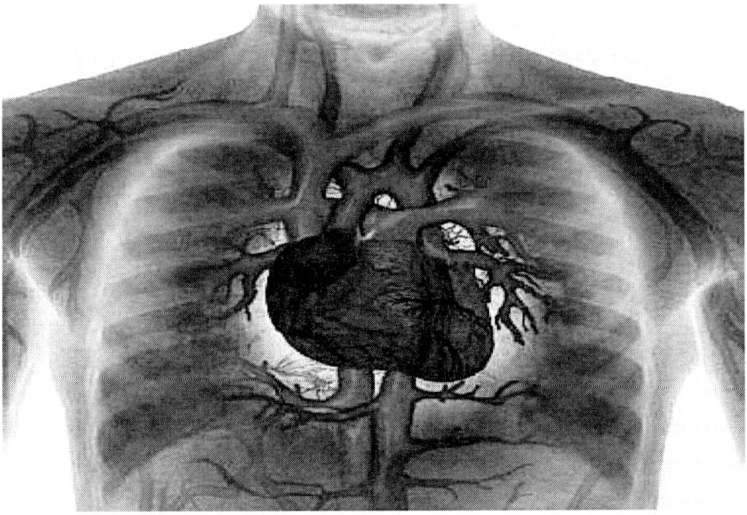

45. Coronary Heart Disease

Heart is one of the most important parts of out body as it controls the blood flow. Not only does it caters to regulation the circulation of the blood, but also maintains the level of purity of our blood. While improper diet is the main cause for heart disease, there are also several other reasons that lead to the occurrence of coronary heart disease. The seven major causes of heart diseases are elevated blood levels of cholesterol, elevated blood pressure, elevated blood uric acid levels, certain metabolic disorders, obesity, smoking and lack of physical exercise. The symptoms of it are shortness of breath, chest pain or pain down arm, palpitations, fatigue, fainting, emotional instability, cold hands and feet. Coronary heart disease has become the major cause of death around the world and needs to be controlled. The best way to deal with this disease would be to retreat to the natural remedies.

Home Remedy for Heart Disease

- A simple yet effective method to treat heart disease would be to drink milk with garlic. Put a clove of garlic in a glassful of milk. Drink this warm milk before going to bed. Do this for a few days.

- For people who have heart pain along with high blood pressure, prepare a soup of the bottle gourd vegetable. Do not put in large amount of spices and oil. Intake this in the morning and evening.
- In 2 tsp of pure ghee, mix 2 milliliters of the juice of the bael fruits (Aegle marmelos). Have this once in a day regularly. This is the best remedy for people who already had one seizure, as it reduces the possibility of the other.
- Prepare a powder using some roasted asafetida. Add equal amounts of Bishop's weed seeds, some rock salt and white or black cumin seeds. Grind this mixture well and store it in a glass bottle. Intake 2 to 3 grams of this powder every day.
- In 100 milliliters of ginger juice, add a little amount of honey. Lick this once a day. It will improve the chest pains.
- Mix equal proportions of powdered pods of a cardamom, root of the banyan tree and leaves of the wild snake gourd. Lick this powder with ghee once a day.
- Take some pomegranate leaves and some water. Grind the leaves in the water and then strain the mix. Drink the strained water. This would cure of all the heart diseases.
- Mix 200 milliliters of fresh carrot juice and100 milliliters of spinach juice. Drink this mixture every day in the morning. Apart from stopping the heart aches, it also reduces the chances of heart attacks.
- A simple way to treat heart disease would be to have an amla every day. Rich in vitamin C, it would prevent any heart disease.
- Consuming a glass of beet juice or fresh grape juice every day reduces the chances of any heart disease.
- In 10 ml of pomegranate juice, add 10 grams of finely ground sugar. Have this during chest congestions and heart aches.

- Intake parsley tea for about 3 to 4 times a day. Since parsley is good in treating heart disease, it would work perfectly, curing any kind of heart pain.
- Have 1 tsp of onion juice first thing in the morning. It would be helpful in normalizing the percentage of blood cholesterol by oxidizing excess cholesterol.
- Increase the consumption of foods rich in Vitamin E & B such as leafy green vegetables, sardines, egg yolks, nuts, yeast, meat, low-fat dairy products and lentils.

46. Heart Palpitation

Heart beats occur at normal pace and are regular in nature. When these become irregular and strong or forceful, they are known as heart palpitations. It has become a common phenomenon and is seen among both men and women of all age groups. Some of the causes for heart palpitations are stress, incorrect diet, and sometimes unhealthy lifestyle. The other reasons for palpitations are nervousness, increased physical activity, flatulence and excessive smoking. Heart palpitations are the first signs that the heart is not in the proper state. The most common symptoms of heart palpitations are an increase in pulse rate and a thumping feeling in the chest.

Home Remedies for Palpitation

- The best way to cure palpitations naturally would be to have a guava empty stomach. Have this in the morning regularly. Not only would it treat palpitations but provide a soothing effect.
- Another remedy would be to have grape juice every day. This would relieve a person suffering from palpitations.
- In a glass of water, add a tablespoon of honey and half cup of lemon juice. Have this combination before going to bed. This is a good remedy to cure heart palpitations.
- Prepare a paste using some snake gourd leaves and water. Put the paste in the cheesecloth and squeeze the juice out of it. Intake this 1 to 2 tablespoon about thrice a day.

- Take some Indian spikenard and add a pinch of camphor and cinnamon. Have this in two to three grams. Another way to have it would be to take it as an infusion in doses of 30 to 60 ml, thrice a day.
- Grind equal amounts of dry coriander, jaggery, and aniseed and make a powdery substance. Have 6 grams of this combination after every meal.
- Increase in the intake of fresh vegetables and fruits. This would relieve a person suffering from heart palpitations.
- Include some physical activities in the regular day to day living. Swimming, cycling and other outdoor sports as your means of exercise are good ways to keep the heart healthy.
- Avoid taking in caffeinated beverages such as soft drinks, alcohol, coffee and tea. These increase the occurrence of heart palpitations.
- Squeeze half of the lemon and mix about 1 tsp of honey to the lime juice. Add 250 ml of water to it. Intake this mixture every day as it would reduce the problem of palpitations.

47. Heartburn

A burning sensation and pain in the stomach and chest region is termed as heartburn. Also known as pyrosis, it is generally a burning or painful sensation in the esophagus. This is caused due to the upward direction of gastric acid from the stomach to the chest. On its way up, the acid aggravates the tissues in the esophagus and the throat. Though termed heartburn, it is a digestive problem and is not concerned with the functioning of the heart. Eating fatty/oily foods, pregnancy, wearing extremely tight clothes, bending down, sleeping on a full stomach are some of the causes of heartburn. The symptoms of heartburn are bloating, gas, nausea, shortness of breath and/or an acidic or sour taste in the throat and mouth. However, heartburn can be treated at home using natural remedies.

Home Remedy for Heartburn

- On the first sign of heartburn, it is advisable to have water in larger quantities. This would work for those, whose symptoms are not too strong.
- An easy home remedy for heartburn would be to have half a tsp of baking soda in a glass of water. It is effective in treating heartburn.
- Combine 1 tablespoonful of apple cider vinegar, 1 teaspoonful of honey and 1 cup of warm water. Having this mixture would provide relief from heartburn.
- Consuming buttermilk during heartburn would bring in relief. It works very well for the ailment.

- Cinnamon is useful in treating heartburn. Make tea using cinnamon sticks. Have this tea once or twice a day. Another way to have it would be to prepare cinnamon sandwich.
- In a cup of water, add 1 ½ tsp of ginger root. Simmer this for about 10 minutes. Intake this drink as it would bring in relief for the pain.
- In a pan of 1 cup boiling water, put a tablespoon of the dried marshmallow root. Cover the pan with a lid and allow it to simmer for 15 minutes. Strain this liquid and have at least 3 - 4 cups per day.
- Drinking Aloe Vera juice acts beneficially in healing intestinal tract and thus relieving a person suffering from heartburn.
- Take 1 or 2 raw potato and wash them well. Do not peel, instead, cut them into pieces and churn them. Drink the juice immediately. The other option would be to mix it with some other juice for taste. However make sure that it is drunk instantly.
- Prepare tea using chamomilc tea. Intake this tea after meals. This would relieve a person from esophageal irritation.
- Take 1 tsp of yellow mustard with about ½ glass of water. This would stop heartburn instantly.
- Take a cabbage and cut it into pieces. Immerse this in a pot of water and let it cook for about 7 minutes. Thereafter, add some mashed potatoes and a little olive oil. Have this mixture. It would heal the sensation of heartburn.

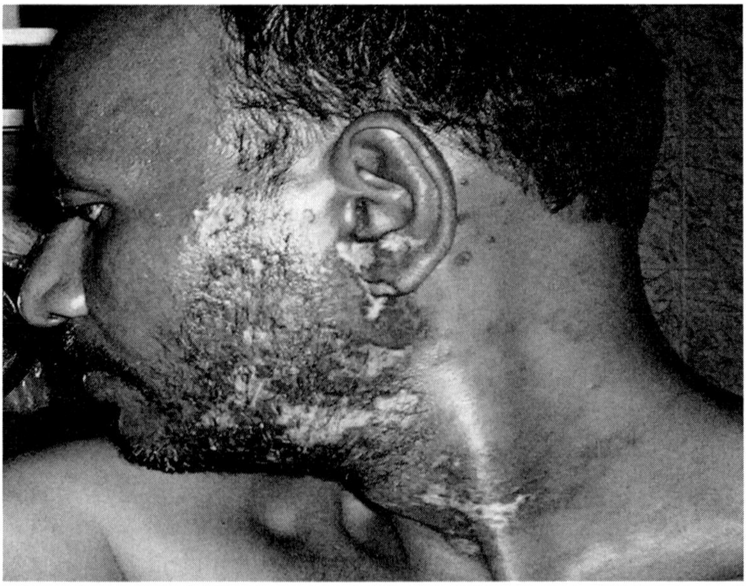

48. Herpes

A highly contagious infection, herpes is a viral infection caused by the herpes simplex virus. There are two types of herpes - oral herpes that causes cold sores or fever blisters around the mouth. The other, genital herpes, causes sores below the waist. The latter is sexually transmitted and causes pain and blisters in the genital area. Herpes can be transferred by kissing, sharing eating utensils or having intimate contact. Stress, fatigue, pregnancy, hormonal imbalance and cosmetic surgery are also some of the causes of herpes. Painful sores, flu-like symptoms, fever, and swollen glands are some of the symptoms of herpes. They might be mild, moderate or even severe. However, herpes can be treated at home naturally.

Home Remedy for Herpes

- The most popular and effective home remedies for herpes is rub ice on the herpes for a few minutes. It would provide instant healing effect.

- Prepare black coffee without sugar. After having the coffee, apply the remains in the cup, on the herpes.
- Take some baking powder and pat a cotton ball with it over the infected area. This would be beneficial in treating herpes.
- Take 5 drops each of Bergamot oil and eucalyptus oil. Coat this mix on the herpes affected area after every few minutes.
- Take a cup of olive oil and pour it in a pot. Add some bee wax and lavender oil to it and cook the mixture. When cooked, allow it to cool. Thereafter, coat it on the herpes.
- In 3 liters of water, add 25 grams each of dried mullein, mallow roots and marsh mallow roots. Simmer it for about 3 minutes. Filter the mixture and use on a compress day and might. This would reduce irritation and also prevent herpes.
- Grate a carrot and wrap it in a cloth. Apply this on the blisters. It would lessen glandular swelling and alleviate the pain, thereby, providing healing effect.
- Increase in the consumption of foods rich in vitamins, zinc and iron. It is also advisable to have lots of leafy vegetables and fruits.
- Take a tea bag and dip it in a cup of hot water. Apply this warm tea bag on the blisters for half an hour.
- Applying Aloe Vera gel on the blisters also provides relief from the herpes.
- Take a cotton ball and dip it in cornstarch. Dab this cotton on the sores. It would provide relief to a person suffering from herpes.
- Intake a cup of peppermint tea as it would be helpful in lessening the pain and fever.

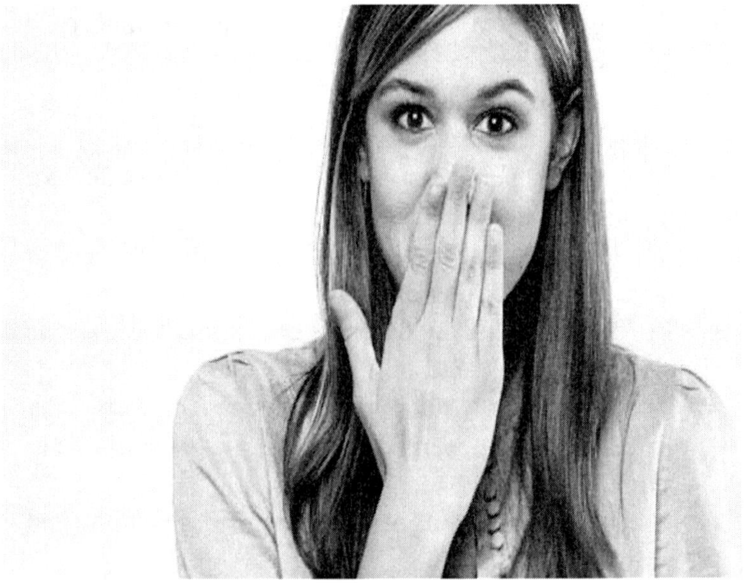

49. Hiccups

Hiccups are involuntary actions over which we have not control. These reflex actions are caused due to the contractions in the diaphragm muscles. The diaphragm muscle divides the chest from the stomach. Hence, irritation in this causes breathing to be erratic, which causes the sound. Other causes of hiccups are eating too much and too fast, sudden excitement, hot and spicy foods, stomach disorders, kidney problems and infection in lungs. Although hiccups disappear on their own, continuous hiccups for a day or two is a cause for concern. Given are some home remedies for hiccups.

Home Remedy for Hiccups

- A simple home remedy for hiccups would be to have water frequently in short durations.
- Having a spoonful of peanut butter would work well in stopping hiccups.

- Taking deep breaths when a person is having hiccups is beneficial.
- A good home remedy for treating hiccups is to gargle, using lukewarm water.
- Lick a tablespoon of sugar slowly. This is an effective natural way to cure hiccups.
- Yet another simple trick would be to divert the mind to something else. this is effective in stopping hiccups.
- In a cup of yoghurt, add 2 tsp of common salt. Have this slowly to stop the hiccups.
- Take 2 cups of water and add ½ tsp of cardamom powder to it. Boil the water and then filter it. Have the filtrate to stop the hiccups.
- Another remedy would be to suck crushed ice. This would provide instant relief.
- Take a piece of ginger and suck it slowly. This would stop the hiccups.
- Combine 1/2 tsp mustard seeds with 1/2 tsp of pure ghee. Swallow this mixture as it would stop the hiccups instantly.

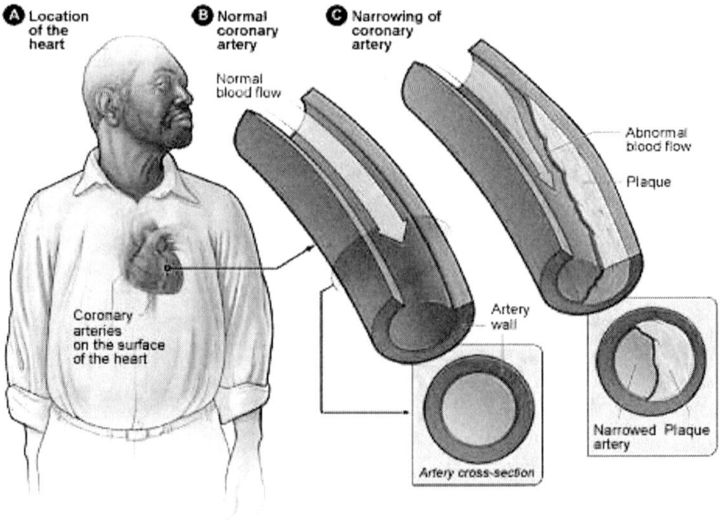

50. High Blood Cholesterol

Cholesterol is one of the important elements in the body. Produced in the liver, it is a yellowish fatty substance which performs functions such as transportation of fat, providing defense mechanism, protecting red blood cells and muscular membrane of the body. Cholesterol is also produced from the food which is consumed. The normal level of cholesterol varies between 150 - 200 mg per 100 ml, an increase in which, results in high cholesterol. The most common symptoms of high blood cholesterol are general fatigue, excess sweating and feel of uneasiness, pain and heaviness in chest area and breathlessness. Excessive smoking and alcohol consumption, eating high fat diet, obesity and heredity factors are some of the causes for high cholesterol. However, high cholesterol can be controlled at home using certain home remedies.

Home Remedy for High Cholesterol

- The best home remedy to cure a person with high cholesterol is to have at least 8-10 glasses of water per day.

- Immerse 2 tablespoons of coriander seeds in a glass of water. Boil the concoction and allow it to cool. Strain the water and have it three times a day.
- Take 10 pieces of cinnamon sticks and put them in a pot containing 5 teacups of water. Boil the water and then add a tablespoon of honey to it. Drink this concoction when it's warm.
- In a glassful of milk, add a piece of garlic and boil it. Allow it to cool before drinking. Consume this for a few days. Not only would it reduce cholesterol, but also take care of the cardiac pains.
- Alternatively, a person who has problems of high cholesterol can also have 2-3 cloves of garlic per day.
- Mix 10-12 tablespoons of apple juice and 5-6 tablespoons of apple cider vinegar. Intake this mixture once a day.
- Consuming raw onions or onion juice is also beneficial in reducing the high cholesterol.
- Regular exercising is very necessary to keep the cholesterol levels under control.
- In green leafy salads, mix a small amount of olive oil. It proves beneficial lessening the high cholesterol levels as well as for the proper functioning of the heart and the body.
- Persons suffering from high cholesterol should have foods rich in fiber such as raspberries, blackberries, strawberries, broccoli, green beans, etc.
- Consume lots of almonds and walnuts. These are helpful in reducing the cholesterol levels.
- Chewing sweet neem is also beneficial in lowering the high cholesterol levels.
- Having fenugreek seeds and sprouts helps to reduce the high cholesterol levels.

- Persons suffering from high cholesterol levels should have a small bowl of curd everyday. Curd acts favorably in reducing the cholesterol levels.
- Another effective natural remedy to treat high cholesterol levels would be to have foods rich in lecithin such as egg yolk, vegetable oils, whole grain cereals, soybeans and un-pasteurized milk.
- It is advisable to have food prepared from sunflower seeds instead of butter and saturated oil. This is highly beneficial in regulating the cholesterol levels.

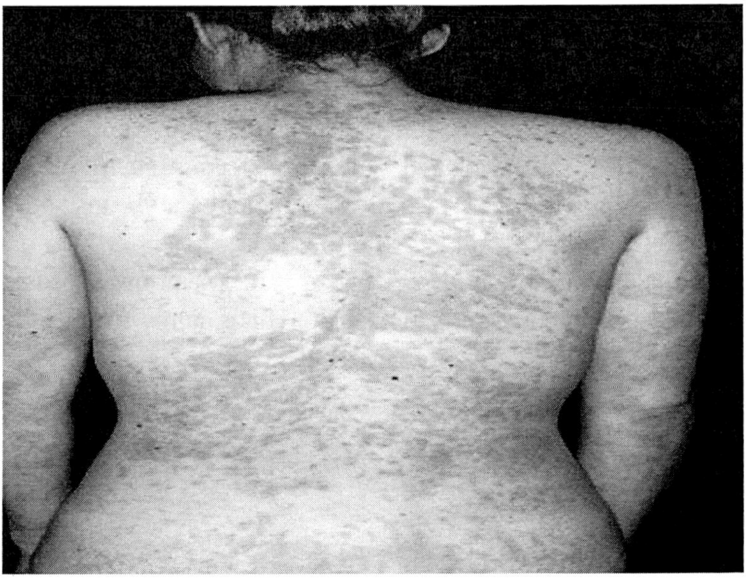

51. Hives

Medically known as urticaria, hives is an ailment of the skin which causes rings and patches all over the body. Hives are caused by a chemical termed as histamine, which is why red blotches form on the skin surface. These appear in groups and are generally red in color. Hives appear in different sizes, varying on how serious the illness is. It is usually caused when a person is allergic to a particular thing. These may be a particular medicine, nuts, eggs, berries, insect bites, jelly fish, etc. at times, it also occurs due to tight clothes, exposure to extreme weather, hereditary or even sweat. The most common symptoms of hives are swelling on the affected region, itchiness, pain and difficulty in doing routine activity. However, hives can be cured at home retreating to the natural remedies.

Home Remedy for Hives

- The most popular and effective way to cure hives would be to ka e cool compresses. Taking cool showers or bath would help in treating hives.

- A natural way to cure hives would be to apply Vitamin E oil on the affected area. Repeat the process at least two times a day.
- Fill half of the bathtub with lukewarm water and add ½ cup each of cornstarch and baking soda. Soak the body in this water. It is an effective remedy for treating hives.
- Drinking peppermint, chamomile or valerian tea is helpful in curing hives. These soothe the mind and are thus helpful in treating hives.
- Coat the affected area with Aloe Vera. This is helpful in curing hives. One can either go for the pulp of Aloe Vera or the cream containing it.
- Prepare tea adding 2 tsp of powdered stinging nettle. To this, add a tsp of honey or a few drops of lemon for flavor. Nettles are known to have healing effect over the hives.
- Increase the consumption of foods that are rich in Vitamin C and Vitamin E with Zinc.
- Mix 2 cups of oatmeal and 3 tsp of cornstarch. Add a little water to make a paste. Coat the hive-affected area with this paste for about half an hour. Then, wash with water.
- Swimming in chlorine water is beneficial in treating hives. It would help to drive out the hives.
- In a tsp of olive oil or vegetable oil, add a few drops of grapefruit seed extract. Apply this mixture over the affected area. This solves dual purpose - reduces itching as well as heals hives.
- Alternatively, add grapefruit seed extract in a cup of water. spray the solution on the affected area.
- Dab milk of magnesia on the affected area. This would remove the irritation as well as the itching. Apply this several times a day.

- It is advisable to avoid any kind of heat in the body. This would dilate the blood vessel and increases the hives instead.
- In a cup of boiling water, add a tablespoon of oatmeal. Allow it to steep for half an hour. Thereafter, strain the mixture and apply it over the affected using a cotton ball.

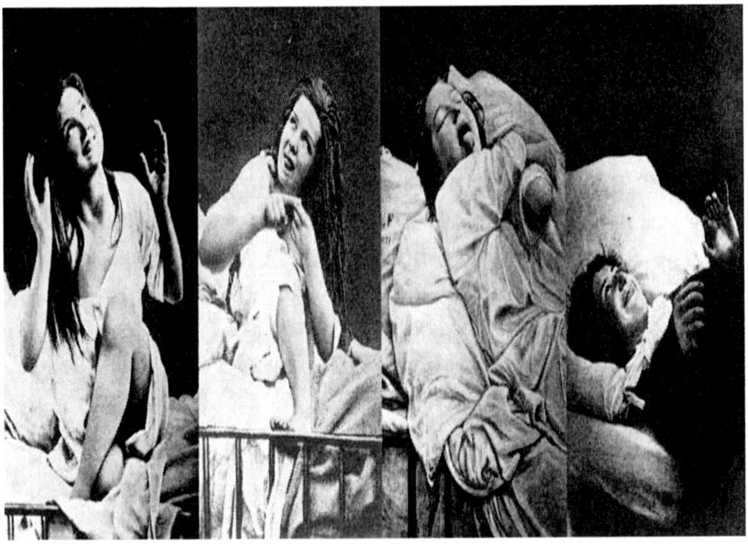

52. Hysteria

Hysteria is a neurological condition which causes mental and nervous disorder. It makes the patient emotionally disturbed as he/she does not have any control over feeling and sentiments. Such patients usually suffer from any phobia, lack of self-discipline, depression and seizures. Some of the causes of hysteria are sexual excess or sexual repression, idleness, hereditary, mental strain, stress, fear, worry, depression, etc. Heavy breathing, clenched teeth, tensing of muscles, swelling of veins particularly in the neck region, alternating bouts of laughter and crying are the most common symptoms of hysteria. Though found in both the sexes, hysteria is more prevalent among females than in males. It usually occurs during adolescence and becomes less frequent after 25 years of age. Treating hysteria at home is the best way to deal with the disorder.

Home Remedy for Hysteria

- An effective way to treat hysteria patients would be to take utmost care of their diet. They should start with a fruit diet for all the three meals such as apples, grapes, oranges, pineapples, papayas, grapefruits, etc. Thereafter, follow an all-milk diet for a month.

- In a cup of freshly made lettuce juice, mix a tsp of Indian gooseberry (amla) juice. Have this mixture in an empty stomach every morning for a month.
- Consuming a tablespoon of honey everyday is beneficial in treating patients suffering from hysteria.
- Make asafetida a part of the regular diet. Include it in small quantity of 0.5 to 1.0 grams per day.
- Alternatively, the patient can also smell some asafetida every day.
- Add a gram of Rauwolfia root in a glass of milk. Intake this milk twice everyday - morning and evening. Drink this combination until completely cured.
- Appropriate sleep and regular exercise is very beneficial in treating patients with hysteria.
- Grate the vegetable bottle Gourd and apply on the forehead of the patient. It is a very good treatment for curing hysteria.

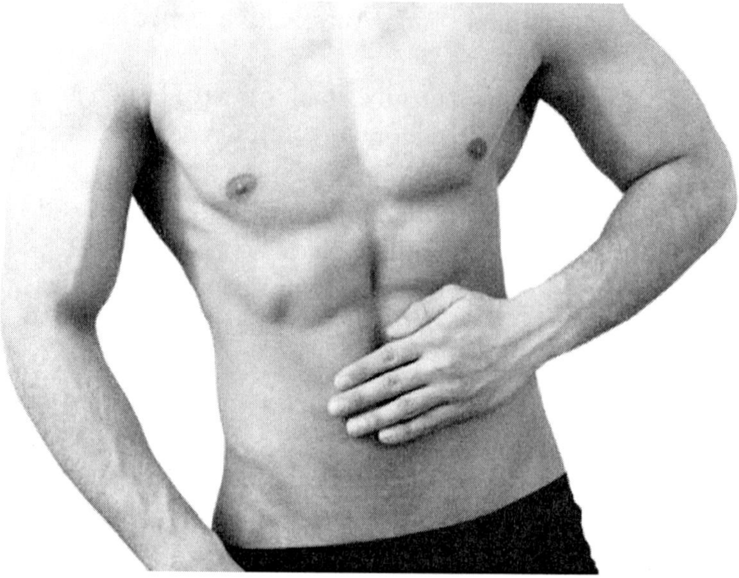

53. Indigestion

Also known as dyspepsia, indigestion is a problem related to the stomach. It occurs when the digestive juices are not secreted properly as such resulting in uneasiness. Consuming a variety of food stuffs is one of the prime reasons for indigestion. Other causes are overeating, eating hurriedly without chewing properly, lack of exercise, improperly cooked food and also food allergies from beans, onions, seafood, etc. indigestion leads to pain in belly, nausea, bloating of stomach, uncontrolled burping, heartburn, flatulence and acid regurgitation. While indigestion occurs to men and women, its occurrence is more in females when compared to males. However, it is not a very serious problem and can be cured retreating to some home remedies.

Home Remedy for Indigestion

- A useful home remedy for treating indigestion would be to have half glass of pineapple juice after meals.
- In a glass of lukewarm water, add a spoonful of juice of lemon, one spoonful of ginger and two spoons of honey.

Mix it well and drink. An effective remedy to cure indigestion.

- In a cup of hot water, mix a tablespoon of lemon juice. Have this mixture before meals. It would prevent any indigestion.
- It is recommended to apply some ice cubes over the stomach after meals. This would cure indigestion.
- Take equal parts of baking soda and water in a glass. Have this mixture. It would provide instant relief from indigestion.
- Add a tsp of cumin seeds in a glass of water. Drink this mixture.
- Consume a gram or two of the pulp of the belleric myrobalan fruit. This would ease and provide relief from indigestion.
- In a tsp of fresh coriander leaf juice, add a pinch of salt. Drink this two times a day.
- Alternatively, 1 or 2 tsp of coriander juice added to freshly prepared buttermilk is also effective in treating indigestion
- Eating half a tsp of aniseed is likely to be effective in treating indigestion.
- Take a tsp of ajwain and add a pinch of rock salt to it. Have this mixture for curing indigestion.
- Another effective remedy would be to chew a small piece of ginger sprinkled with salt for 5 to 10 minutes before meals.
- Intake a tablespoon of cinnamon water after one hour of having meals proves helpful in treating digestion problem.
- Consume 1 cup of ginger tea after food to solve the problem of indigestion.
- Having oranges and grapes would serve beneficially in curing indigestion.

- Add 2 to 3 drops of mint essence in a glass of water. have this concoction every 3 to 4 hours to get relieved from indigestion.
- Take half a cup of Soya oil and add 2 to 3 drops of garlic oil. Massaging the stomach with this mixture is likely to bring relief from digestion problems.
- Prepare herbal tea using blackberry, raspberry, mint and chamomile. This would be useful in curing indigestion.
- Add a few drops of lemon or cider vinegar in a glass of water. Drink this mixture before meals.
- Consume a mixture of 1 tsp each of mint juice, lemon juice, and honey. This is effective in treating indigestion.

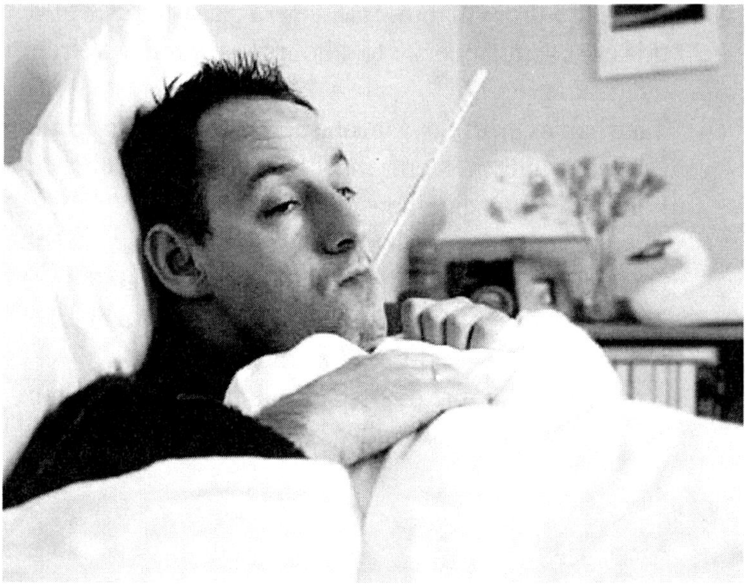

54. Influenza

Influenza or more popularly known as flu is a highly contagious disease. It is caused due to infection from influenza viruses. Flu generally affects the like nose, ear, eyes, throat and lungs spreading to the lungs and the bronchi. Striking suddenly, influenza has the capability to spread like an epidemic engulfing a large portion of the population. Chills, fever, headache and severe muscular pains are the starting symptoms of influenza. Some of the causes of influenza are viral infection, unhealthy lifestyle, tension and stress, excessive workload, lack of proper exercise, living in stuffy rooms and staying awake up till late hours. There is no proper medication for flu. Nonetheless, it can be treated using natural remedies.

Home Remedy for Influenza

- The best remedy to cure influenza would be to have plenty of fluids. Do not let the body get dehydrated as liquids thin all the nasal secretion.

- Dip a cloth with cold water and apply it on the forehead. This would be effective in curing influenza.
- In a cup of boiling water add, 1 tsp bayberry bark, 1 tsp grated ginger root and ½ tsp cayenne powder. Allow it to sit for about 20 minutes before drinking. This is an effective way to cure influenza.
- Increase in the consumption of foods rich in vitamin C. this is because it gives a boost to the immune system and increases the white blood cells.
- Include garlic in the diet. Eat raw garlic empty stomach in the morning.
- A simple way to get relieved from flu would be to have bath in tub to lukewarm water.
- Ginger tea is helpful in curing flu. Prepare a tea by adding 2-3 slices of ginger.
- Alternatively, instead of ginger, garlic can also be used. Make tea using 2-3 cloves of garlic.
- Combine ½ tsp of powdered long pepper, two teaspoons of honey and ½ tsp of ginger juice. Have this combination three times a day.
- In a cup of warm milk, add a tsp of turmeric. Intake such milk, thrice a day. Not only would it prevent complications arising from influenza, it would also activate the liver.
- Mix equal amounts of onion juice and honey. Consume 3 to 4 tsp of this mixture everyday.
- Prepare fenugreek decoction by boiling one tablespoon of fenugreek seeds in ½ liter of water, till it is reduced to 1/3rd. In a cup of this fenugreek decoction, add a tsp of fresh ginger juice and honey to flavor. Intake this mixture.
- Intake grapefruit juice as it helps in treating influenza.
- In ½ liter of water, add one gram of holy basil leaves along with some ginger. Boil this decoction until only ½ the mixture is left. Have this decoction as tea.

- Warm some water and mix a few drops of lemon and some honey. This is a good mixture to loosen phlegm.
- For the non-vegetarians, consume chicken soup as it is useful in treating influenza.

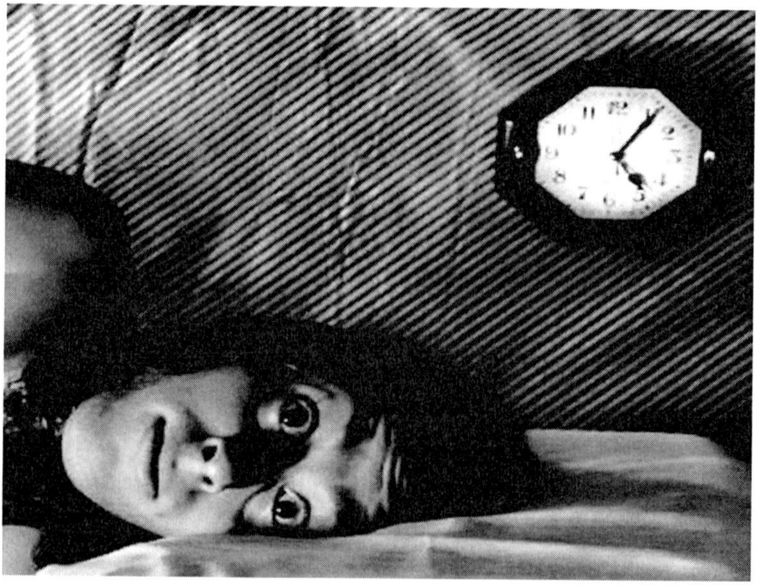

55. Insomnia

Insomnia is referred to the inability to sleep. It is a condition when a person faces difficulty in sleeping at night. Sleepless nights are a worrisome issue and affect the day-to-day work. The major symptoms of insomnia are difficulty in falling asleep/ staying asleep, waking up during the night, inability to fall back to sleep when awakened in the middle of the night and inability to sleep during regular hours. For some people the problem is such that they need to take sleeping pills every night to get some rest. Tension, anxiety, stress, suppressed resentment, anger, bitterness, constipation, overeating, excessive tea/coffee/smoking are some of the causes sleeplessness. Insomnia can, however, be cured using some natural remedies.

Home Remedy for Insomnia

- An effective way to treat insomnia would be to have milk form the poppy seeds. Extract 30 grams of milk from poppy seeds and add some sugar to it. Have this mixture everyday after dinner.

- Grind four nutmegs to make a fine powder out of it. Have this powder every night before going to sleep.
- Insomnia can be treated following the same routine i.e. try to sleep at a fixed time every night and wake up at a fixed time in the morning. This would set a sleeping schedule.
- Hot fomentations help to solve the problem of insomnia. Apply hot packs to the spine and have hot footbath before going to bed.
- Intake a cup of milk with honey. This is effective in curing insomnia.
- Grind the root of pippali (Piper longum) plant to make a fine powder. Every night, have 1 tsp of this powder along with jaggery and a glass of warm milk.
- Take a ripe banana and mash it. Add roasted cumin seeds to it and mix properly. Consume this mashed mix before going to sleep.
- Extract fresh juice of valerian wallichi. Intake 1 tsp of this every night before going to sleep.
- Do regular exercise or partake in some physical activities everyday. This would /solve the problem of insomnia. Walking, jogging, skipping and swimming are the good exercises for treating insomnia.
- Mix 1 tsp each of juice of celery leaves with stalks and honey. Consume this mixture everyday.
- Consuming raw onion salad everyday can solve the problem of sleep.
- Combine 2 tsp of fenugreek leaves juice with 1 tsp of honey. Have this combination at bed times daily.
- It is advisable to have 3 cups of curd everyday for people suffering from lack of sleep.
- In a cup of boiling water, add 1 tsp each of chamomile flowers, hops and valeria. Let it steep for 45. Thereafter, strain the drink and have it an hour before sleeping.

- Combine bottle gourd juice and sesame oil in equal parts. Massage this combination on the scalp every night.
- Alternatively, cooked leaves of the bottle gourd can be taken as a vegetable. This is also helpful in curing insomnia.
- Increase in the consumption of vitamin B foods such as wholegrain cereals, pulses, and nuts. These are effective in treating insomnia.
- In half a liter of water, ad one tablespoon of lettuce seeds. Boil this concoction until it reduces to 1/3rd quantity. Have this decoction when warm.
- Boil 375 ml of water. Add a tsp of aniseed and cover the lid of the pan. Let it simmer for 15 minutes. Strain the decoction and drink when warm. Hot milk and honey can also be added to the tea.
- Mix 0.25 gm to 0.5 gm of rauwolfia with some scented substance like cardamom. If the problem is chronic, double the intake, one in the morning and one in the evening.

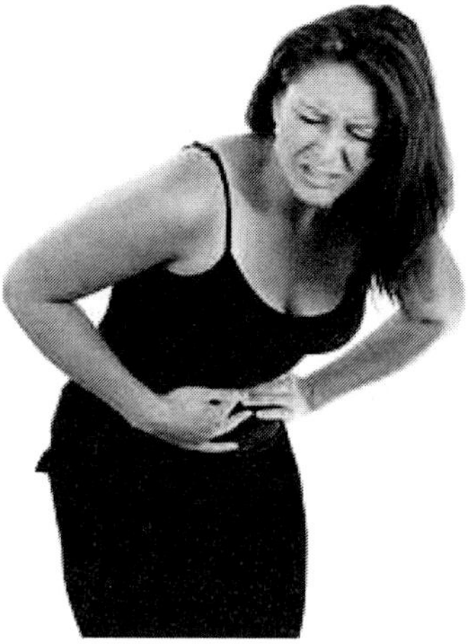

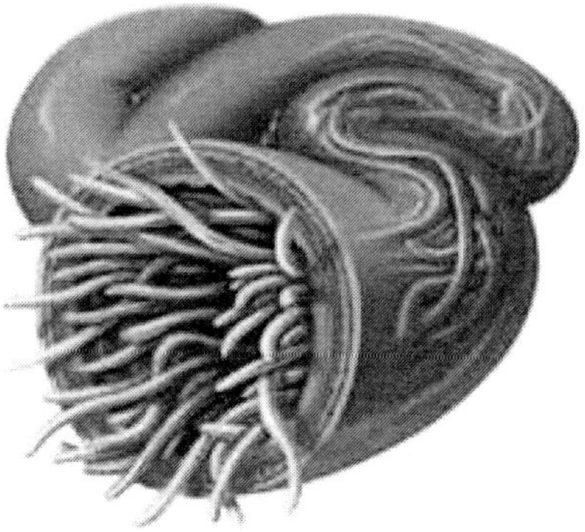

56. Intestinal Worms

The human body especially the stomach and the intestine is home to a number of parasites such as hookworms, roundworms, flatworms, etc. These parasites are helpful in the digestive process. However, at times, the parasites also create several problems. there are various causes for the problems caused - contaminated food, dirty fingers and food, faulty living, etc. some of the symptoms observed in people suffering from intestinal worms are diarrhea, foul breath, dark circles under the eyes, inflammation of the intestine and lungs, nausea, vomiting, anaemia and nutritional disorders, constipation and loss of weight. Intestinal worms can, nonetheless, be treated at home.

Home Remedy for Intestinal Worms

- Ground some coconut and store it. Every morning, take a tablespoon of coconut at the breakfast. After three hours, take 30 to 60 ml of castor oil mixed with 250 to 375 ml of lukewarm milk. Repeat the process for a few days.

- Chewing three cloves of garlic every morning is likely to relieve a person suffering from intestinal worms.
- Grate a small cup of carrot. Have this early in the morning on an empty stomach. This is an effective way to treat intestinal worms.
- Extract fresh juice from an unripe papaya. Mix A tablespoon of this juice with three to four tablespoons of hot water. after two hours, have 30 to 60 ml of castor oil mixed in 250-375 ml of lukewarm milk. Repeat this for two days.
- Papaya seeds are also useful in treating intestinal worms. Powder the seeds and take 1 tsp of it with a cup of milk or water first thing in the morning.
- Papaya leaves are also beneficial in curing intestinal worms. Pour 250 ml of boiling water in a pan containing 15 gm of dry papaya leaves. Take this decoction with honey.
- Cut the bark of the pomegranate tree. Make a cold decoction of it and have it in the quantity of 90 to 180 ml three times a day. A purgative should be given after the last dose. For children, the quantity of this decoction is less - 30 to 60 ml.
- Take 1 tablespoon of a ripe pumpkin seeds. Before immersing in 250 ml of boiling water, peel and crush them.
- Powder the herb of wormwood and consume it in a dose of eight to sixteen gram doses daily. This is effective in treating in intestine worms.
- The oil of wormwood is also beneficial. Mix it with olive oil in the ratio of 1:8. Intake this in dose 50 to 100 ml.
- Alternatively, wormwood oil can be mixed with water for treating intestinal worms. In 120 ml of water, add 2 ml of

wormwood oil. Give it as an enema for killing worms in the rectum.

- Mix equal proportions of the herb belleric myroblan and the seeds of the herb butea (palas). Have 1 tsp of this mixture 3 times a day.
- Consume 1 tsp of powdered seeds of butea every day to cure intestinal worms.
- Alternatively, the powdered seeds of butea can also be consumed in the form of a paste. Take 1 tsp each of powdered seeds of butea and honey and make a paste. Have this 3 times a day.
- Take the roots and bark of the vasaka tree. Prepare a decoction taking 30 gm of the root and bark in 500 ml of water. Boil this till the quantity reduces to 1/3rd. have 30 ml of this decoction two times a day for 2-3 days.
- A simple natural remedy would be to have a glass of boiled water with a tablespoon of rock salt. Have this empty stomach every morning.

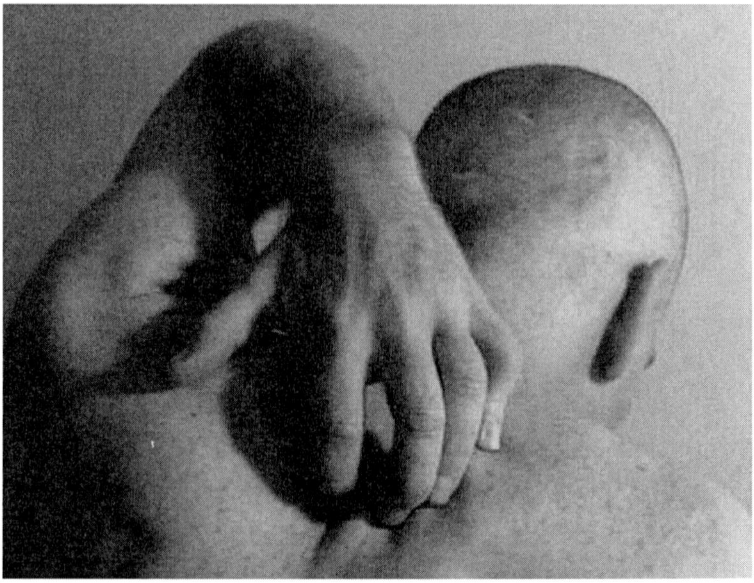

57. Itching

Itching is the irritation of the skin. There is a yearning to scratch the affected area. Almost everybody meets up with this disease at one point of life. Scratching the affected area can create further problems as the skin might get bruised and sore. It can even be painful at the later stages. There are various causes for itching. Dry skin is one of the prime causes for itching. Others include exposure or contact with chemicals, sunburn, cold weather, overexposure to water, insect bites or stings and hot baths. From being limited to a specific area, to being generalized, itching can occur at any part of the body. The desire to scratch the affected area is the symptoms of itching. The best way to deal with it would be to retreat to the natural remedies.

Home Remedy for Itching

- A simple way to treat itching would be to have bath putting 2 cups of oatmeal in a tub with lukewarm water.

- Dust the affected area with cornstarch. Alternatively, some cornstarch can be poured in the bath water as well.
- In the bath water, add 2 tablespoons of apple cider vinegar. This would work well to provide relieve from itching.
- Apply cold compress to the affected area. This is likely to reduce the itchiness caused.
- A good remedy to get relieved from itchiness would be to apply fresh stinging nettle oil on the affected area. Otherwise, drink 1 to 2 cups of Nettle tea daily. For this, add 1 tsp of the dried nettle leaves in a cup of boiling water. Allow it to steep for 15 minutes.
- Soak 2 large handfuls of fresh chickweed in water. When the plant softens, cool it and apply on the affected area.
- Taking bath with lukewarm water is also beneficial in treating the problem of itching.
- Include foods rich in Vitamin C, beta-carotene, Vitamin E and zinc in the diet.
- Take honey and cinnamon powder in equal proportions. Make a fine paste out of it and apply this on the affected area. This would stop itching.
- In a bathtub filled with water, add a cup of white vinegar. Soak the body for 5 to 10 minutes.
- Coat the affected area with a light paste of coconut oil and limejuice. This is a good remedy to cure itching.
- Mix some baking soda with water. make a paste and apply this on the affected area.
- Neem is very useful in treating itchiness. Boil some neem leaves and pour the decoction in the boiling water. Applying neem oil on the affected area is also helpful.

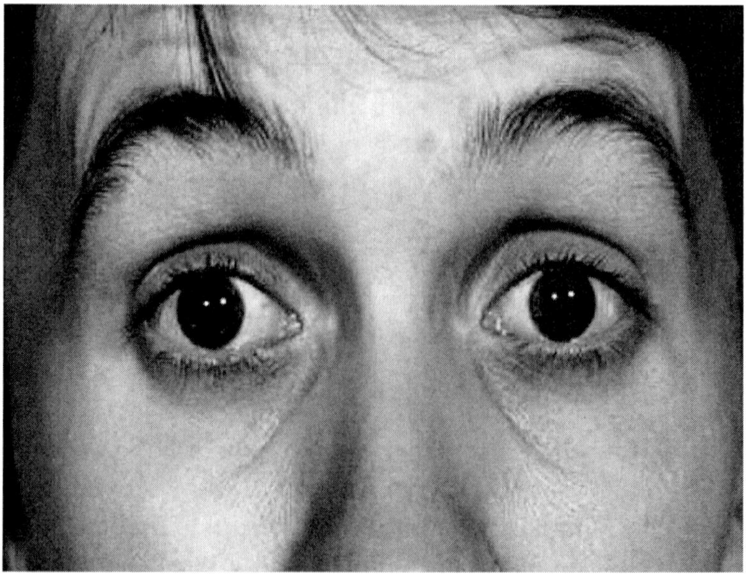

58. Jaundice

One of the most popular liver disorder, jaundice results in the yellowing of skin and whitening of the eyes. It is a condition caused by high-level of pigment bilirubin in the body. The major causes for jaundice are hemolytic anemia, blockage in the bile ducts, acute hepatitis, pancreatic cancer and alcoholic liver disease. Extreme weakness, headache, fever and a dull pain in the liver region are some of the symptoms for jaundice. Bile, a digestive fluid, is essential for nutrition. When prevented from entering the intestine, it results in the increase in gases. Jaundice can, however, be dealt with using some home remedies.

Home Remedy for Jaundice

- Extract the juice of bitter luffa by pounding and squeezing through a cloth. Take the juice on the palm and slowly sniff it. The juice should be drawn through the nostrils.

- The green leaves of the radish are also an effective home remedy. Pound the leaves and extract the juice from them. Intake at least one pound of this juice daily.
- Another effective remedy would be to mash a banana and add to it a tablespoon of honey. Have this mixture two times a day.
- In a glass of buttermilk, mix a pinch of black pepper. Intake this for about a week.
- Take 4 grams of Indian gooseberry with a glass of water. Have this thrice a day for about 20 days.
- In a cup of boiling water, add 8-10 lemon leaves. Cover it with a lid for about 5 minutes. Now, strain the liquid and drink it. Repeat this for 4-5 days.
- Take a cup of water and boil it. To this, add 2 teaspoons of oregano and leave it for 10 minutes. Filter the solution and have it.
- In a glass of buttermilk, add a pinch of roasted alum. Have this 2-3 times a day, regularly.
- Mix 1/4 tsp of turmeric powder in a glass of hot water. Have this 2 to 3 times a day.
- Take tender papaya leaves and make a paste out of it. Consume ½ tsp of this paste with 1 tsp honey.
- Consuming lots of lime juice is beneficial for a person suffering from jaundice.
- Mix 1/2 tsp ginger juice and 1 tsp each of mint juice and lime juice. have this mixture after a span of few hours.
- Have a glass of tomato juice early in the morning. Add some salt and pepper to it, before drinking.
- Squeeze half a lemon in half a cup of beetroot juice. This is an effective remedy for treating jaundice.
- Consuming a glass of carrot juice every day is also beneficial in curing carrot juice.
- Avoid having oils, fried foods, butter, turmeric, spicy food, pickles and sour products.

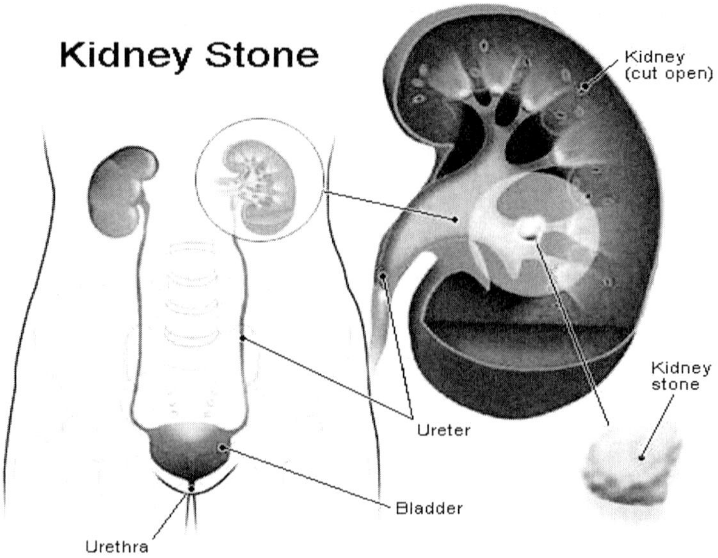

59. Kidney Stones

Kidney stones, which are small, crystallized substances, such as calcium, that form in the kidney or other parts of the urinary tract. Smaller kidney stones can pass out of the body on their own, although this can be painful. Larger stones may require surgery, or they may be broken into smaller pieces with sound waves in a procedure called ultrasonic lithotripsy. Kidney Stones home remedy treatment is quite effective.

Home Remedy for Kidney Stones

- Prepare a potion by boiling two figs in a cup of water. Drink this on an empty stomach in the morning for one month.
- Mix 1 tsp of the juice of Holy basil leaves and 1 tsp of honey. Take this every morning for 5-6 months.
- Eat Watermelon as a fruit or have its juice.

- Take out juice of radish leaves. Take 1 cup of this juice 2 times a day.
- Drink 1 glass of fresh Tomato juice, with a pinch of salt and pepper, empty stomach in the morning.
- Eat 2-3 Apples a day.

60. Leg Cramps

Leg cramps is the term used in reference to a state where a muscle of the leg gets contracted, thereby causing pain and uneasiness. Though leg cramps can affect any person, it occurs more in elderly people. The calf muscle, hamstring and quadriceps are the areas most susceptible to leg cramps. Some of the causes for leg cramps are dehydration, rigorous exercises, muscle fatigue due to overexertion, overweight, fluid imbalances, diminished blood supply and nerve abnormalities. Severe leg pain, muscle tenderness and inability to move the leg are some of the symptoms seen when a person is suffering from leg cramps.

Home Remedies for Leg Cramps

- A glass of lukewarm milk before going to bed is a simple, yet effective way to treat the leg cramps.
- Prepare chamomile tea and have it at least 5 times a day, for about 2 weeks. For every cup of water, take two or three teaspoons of chamomile flower. Bring the water to a boil and let the flower steep in it for a few minutes. Strain, add sugar or honey, and drink warm.
- A hot shower before going to bed is effective in curing leg cramps. Pour some hot water on the painful area as well.
- While you are on bed, stretch the legs as far as you can and keep it in the same position for half an hour. While standing, push your heel onto the floor and bend your toes upwards. This is a good way to treat leg cramps.

- For people who often face the problem of leg cramps, press your toes against the wall and stretch the calf muscles. Repeat this 15-20 times.
- A cup of red raspberry leaf tea, consumed in the morning and evening, is good for relieving a person suffering from leg cramps. Bring a cup of water to a boil and add a tsp red raspberry tea to it. Let it steep for a few minutes, strain and drink when still warm.
- Mix one tbsp of calcium lactate, one tsp of apple cider vinegar and one tsp of honey in half a glass of lukewarm water. Have this once a day. It will be helpful in treating leg cramps.
- Using hot water bottle on the affected area is also beneficial in treating and curing cramps.
- Consume 2-3 bananas per day, as it increases the potassium intake in the body, thereby relieving a person from cramps.
- Having 2 tsp of honey per day is helpful in preventing leg cramps.
- Increase the intake of foods rich in calcium, potassium and magnesium daily.
- Massaging the affected area with essential oils, like lavender oil and rosemary oil and eucalyptus oil. After massaging, wrap the affected area with a towel dipped in hot water.

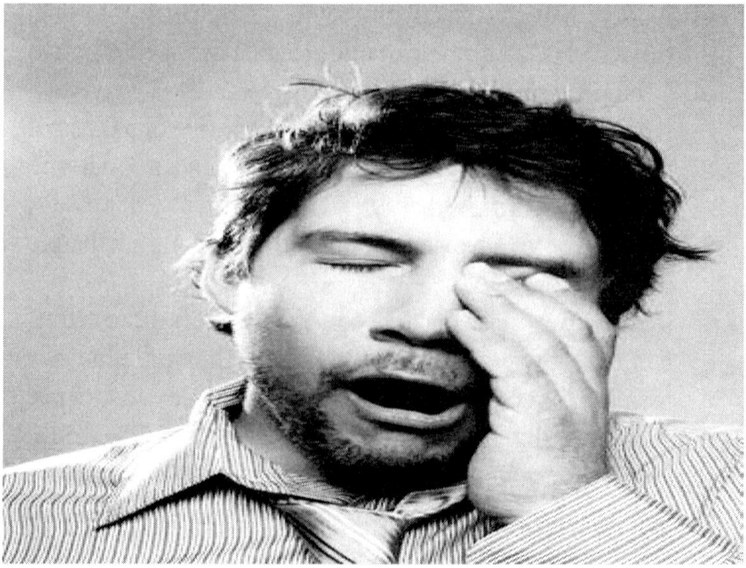

61. Lethargy

Lethargy is a condition that makes a person feel sluggish, drowsy and tired. In such a state, a person feels least interested in his surroundings, in inactive, displays low energy level and carries an attitude of indifference. Some of the symptoms in a lethargic person are change in appetite and bowel movements, pain in different parts of the body, difficulty in doing daily work, fatigue, low concentration and difficulty in falling asleep. Depression is one of the main causes for lethargy. Other causes include high blood pressure, low blood pressure, diabetes, measles, constipation, adrenal gland disorders, thyroid gland disorders and overdose of drugs or alcohol. Lethargy, however, can be treated at home.

Home Remedy for Lethargy

- The most effective home remedy for treating lethargy will comprise of a tea made from holy basil leaves. Put 10 leaves in a cup of water and bring it to a boil. Strain this mixture and have it when warm, not boiling hot.

- A hot bath will be effective in putting off the lethargic feeling.
- Have a glass of grapefruit juice regularly. It will prove to be helpful in treating lethargy.
- Another effective remedy would comprise of a glass of fresh lime juice, to be had every day. It is a good home remedy for curing lethargy.
- Tea and coffee are also beneficial in energizing a lethargic person.
- Regularly exercise makes a person physically more active. It is a great way to rid oneself of the feeling of lethargy.
- Increase the consumption of fruits, vegetables and grains, such as millet, to keep the body well hydrated. It would help revive your spirits.
- Going on a sprout diet for two days in a month is effective in getting over the feeling of lethargy.
- Massaging the body with essential oils, such as rosemary oil and eucalyptus oil, is useful in treating lethargy.
- At times, people feel lethargic when they are involved in uninteresting things. So, it is advisable to invest your time in doing those things in which you have an interest.
- Avoid consuming processed or canned food. Cold beverages like soda and heavy drinks such as rich cream milk should also be avoided.
- Have a balanced diet and include lots of fruits, vegetables and grains in your daily food consumption.

62. Leucoderma

Leucoderma is a condition in which the skin layers experience loss of skin-pigment. Also known as vitiligo, leucoderma causes white patches on the skin surface. It is more common in women than in men and is mostly seen on the hands, neck, back and wrist. The main causes for leucoderma are excessive mental worry and chronic or acute gastric disorders. Other causes involve impaired hepatic function such as jaundice, worms or other parasites in the alimentary canal, typhoid, a defective perspiratory mechanism and burn injuries. It can also be the result of hereditary reasons. However, leucoderma can be treated using certain home remedies, some of which have been mentioned below.

Home Remedies for Leucoderma

- Take about 25 grams of radish seeds and ground them into a powdery substance. Add 2 tsp vinegar and make a fine paste. Apply this paste on the affected area and wash off when dry.
- In about eight liters of water, soak 500 gm turmeric. Boil the concoction until only a liter of it is left. Strain this liquid and add ½ liter mustard oil to it. Apply this on the patchy areas two times a day, for at least 2-3 months.
- Soak psoralea seeds in ginger juice for 3 days. Thereafter, dry them and grind to make a fine powder. Have 1 gram of this powder, with a glass of milk, for about a month. You can also apply this powder on white patches.

- Another method would be to soak psoralea and tamarind seeds in water for 3-4 days. Dry them well and grind to form a paste. Apply this paste on the affected area on a daily basis.
- Goosefoot vegetable is effective in treating leucoderma. Apply the juice of this vegetable on the affected area, once a day. Continue it for 2 months.
- Mix red clay and ginger in equal parts. Apply this on the affected area and wash off when dry.
- Fill a copper vessel with drinking water and leave it overnight. Have this water, on an empty stomach, every morning. This is effective in healing leucoderma.
- Combine 100 gm each of alfalfa and cucumber juice. Consume this mixture two times a day i.e. in the morning and evening. This is a useful home remedy for treating leucoderma.
- Take a handful of dry pomegranate leaves and grind them into a fine powder. Have about 8 grams of this powder every morning and evening, with a glass of water.
- Neem is very effective in treating leucoderma. Try to drink a glass of neem juice everyday.
- Grind black gram and add water, to form a paste. Apply this paste on the affected area, washing off after it dries, for about 4 to 5 months. It is an effective remedy for treating leucoderma.
- Holy basil leaves prove to be beneficial in treating white patches. Consume raw basil leaves or make a decoction out of Holy basil's leaves and stem, along with water.
- Make a poultice of ginger leaves and apply it on the white patches. It is quite effective in treating leucoderma.
- Increase the consumption of walnuts and figs. While walnuts purify blood, figs have healing properties to cure leucoderma.

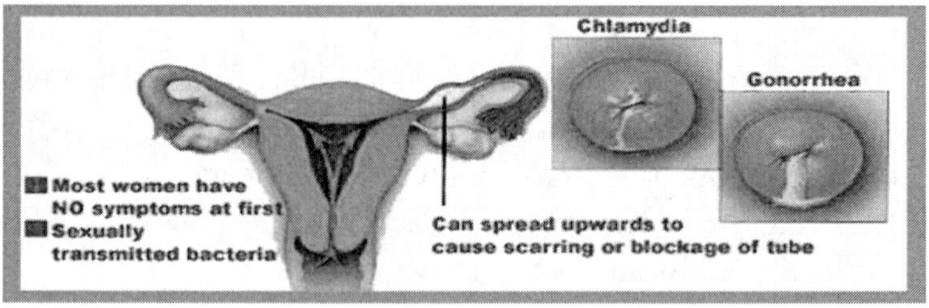

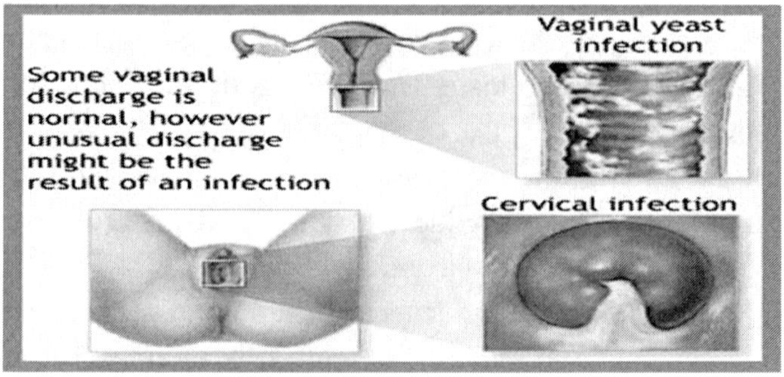

63. Leucorrhoea

Leucorrhea, more popularly known as whites, is a condition that occurs only in females. It is characterized by a white discharge from the genitals. Leucorrhea can lasts from a few days to a few months. However, if not treated at the initial stages, the condition can become chronic. Some of the causes of leucorrhoea include toxicity in the body, thickening of mucous membrane in young women, sexually transmitted diseases, infection occurring during child birth, unhealthy eating habits and maintaining unhygienic conditions (attracting bacteria). While white discharge is main the symptom of Leucorrhea, other symptoms include fatigue, headaches, pain in the lumbar region and the calves and constipation.

Home Remedy for Leucorrhea

- Prepare a paste from the pulp of mango and apply it on the vagina. This is one of the most effective remedies for treating leucorrhea.

- Take 2 to 3 tsp fenugreek seeds and put them in a liter of water. Boil the decoction for about half an hour, on a low flame. Thereafter, strain the mixture and drink it.
- Cook some rice in half a liter of water. Once cooked, strain the water and add a tsp of sugar to it. Drink this liquid. It is useful for treating leucorrhea.
- In one liter of water, put 200 grams ladyfinger. Boil this decoction until the water reduces to half. Strain the mixture and add sugar to taste. Drink 70 ml of this decoction, every 3 hours.
- Put some walnut tree leaves in one liter of water and boil until the mixture is reduced to half. Use it on the affected area, with the help of a douche.
- Soak a tsp of coriander seeds in a glass of water. Keep this overnight and have it, first thing in the morning. Repeat this for a week.
- Chewing betel nut after meals is believed to be helpful in treating leucorrhea.
- Put some guava leaves in one liter of water and boil until the mixture is reduced to half. Use it on the affected area, with the help of a douche.
- Rub either the roof or the leaves of Amaranth in a cup of water. Filter this water and have it two times a day.
- Have 2 grams of Amalaki powder, with sugar or honey. It is effective in curing leucorrhea.
- Consume cranberry juice everyday, as it is believed to be beneficial in treating leucorrhea.
- Consume banana two times a day. Having betel nut, crushed with rose petals and sugar, is also said to be good for treating leucorrhea.

64. Low Blood Pressure

Our body has a definite blood pressure. A drop in the said pressure is a condition termed as hypotension, more popularly low blood pressure. In such a condition, the heart forces the blood out of the arteries with much less strength than it should. Low blood pressure is an outcome of weakened and devitalized system. Some of the main causes of low blood pressure are faulty nutrition or malnutrition, emotional instability, loss of blood and slow internal bleeding. Lethargy, weakness, fatigue and dizziness are the most common symptoms of low blood pressure. A person might even faint, if the arterial pressure gets extremely low. Low blood pressure can, however, be treated naturally, using some home remedies.

Home Remedy for Low Blood Pressure

- The best and the most effective home remedy for treating low blood pressure would be to consume lots of water. This is because dehydration reduces blood volume and leads to a drop in the blood pressure.
- Beetroot juice is beneficial for those suffering from low blood pressure. So, have a cup of raw beetroot juice two times a day.
- Prepare a cup of strong black coffee and consume this whenever you feel that your blood pressure is dipping.
- Put 15-20 gm of Indian Spikenard in 250 ml water and boil it. Now, remove from heat and let it cool down. Have this infusion thrice a day. You can also have 30-40 grains

of Indian Spikenard, along with some camphor and cinnamon.

- Fill your bathtub with lukewarm water and add one kg of Epsom salt to it. Immerse yourself in the bath for 20 minutes, before going to bed. Take caution not to expose the body to a cold area after this.
- In a bowl of water, soak 7 almonds and keep them overnight. Peel them and prepare a paste. Add this paste to lukewarm milk and drink it.
- Take a bowl of water and soak 30 raisins in it, overnight. Chew them one by one, on an empty stomach, in the morning and have water.
- Holy basil works effectively in curing low blood pressure. Take about 15 holy basil leaves and crush them. Filter the mixture with the help of a muslin cloth. Have this filtered mixture, along with a tsp of honey, on an empty stomach.
- Include salt, asafetida and fruits in your diet. All these are beneficial in restoring the blood pressure level.
- Foods rich in proteins, vitamin C and vitamin B are effective in treating low blood pressure.
- Exercises, light walking, swimming and cycling are beneficial in regulating the blood pressure level.

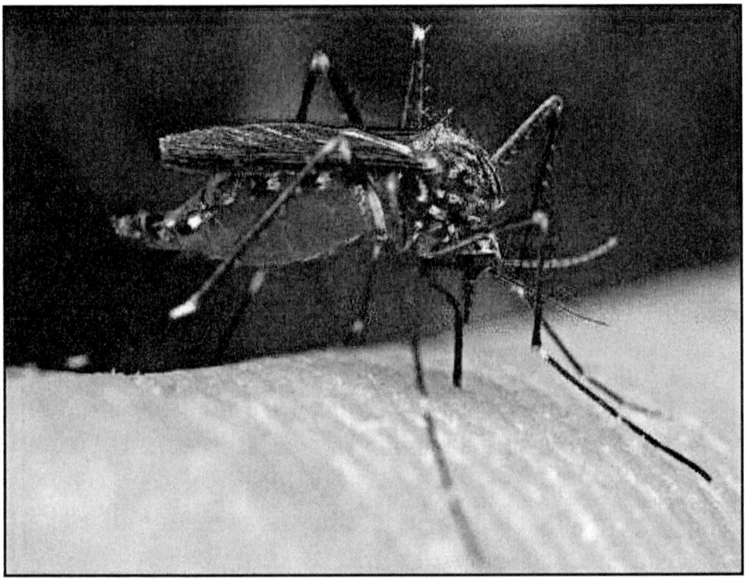

65. Malaria

Malaria is one of the most common diseases found in the tropical and sub-tropical regions. It is basically caused by protozoan parasites of the genus Plasmodium. It is the female Anopheles mosquito that carries the malarial parasites. When it bites a person, the parasites enter the body, wherein they multiply and spread. Malaria mostly affects people with weak immune system or those living in unhealthy living conditions. The most common symptoms of malaria include high fever - accompanied by chills, headache and shivering. Malaria may also result in other complications, such as anemia, kidney failure and dysentery. Here we have provided some home remedies for treating malaria.

Home Remedy for Malaria

- In a glass of water, add a tsp of cinnamon powder, a tsp of honey and a dash of pepper powder. Boil this concoction and have it after it cools down a bit. This is beneficial in treating malaria.

- Dhatura, an Indian herb, is beneficial in treating malaria. Take two and a half freshly sprouted leaves of Dhatura and rub them with jaggery. Convert this mixture into a pill and have it on a daily basis.
- In 60ml of water, dissolve 3 gram of lime and the juice of 1 lemon. Start consuming this, once in a day, right from the time of the onset of fever.
- Roast alum over a hot plate and then powder it. Take a tsp of it when you still have fever. It is a useful remedy for curing malaria.
- Holy basil leaves proves beneficial in treating malaria. You can consume the leaves raw or make a decoction of them and then drink it.
- If the malaria is in the initial stages, an orange juice and water diet can help treat it.
- For the fever in malaria, applying a cold pack on the forehead proves to be beneficial.
- In 250 ml of water, add 15 gm Chirayita herb, along with some cloves or cinnamon. Have 15-30 ml of this solution once in a day, for 15-25 days.
- In a glass of water, put a small piece of ginger and 2-3 teaspoon raisins. Boil this decoction until it gets reduced to half its quantity. Cool down the decoction and consume.
- Avoid junk food, packed food as well as spicy and oily food. It would work to your detriment.

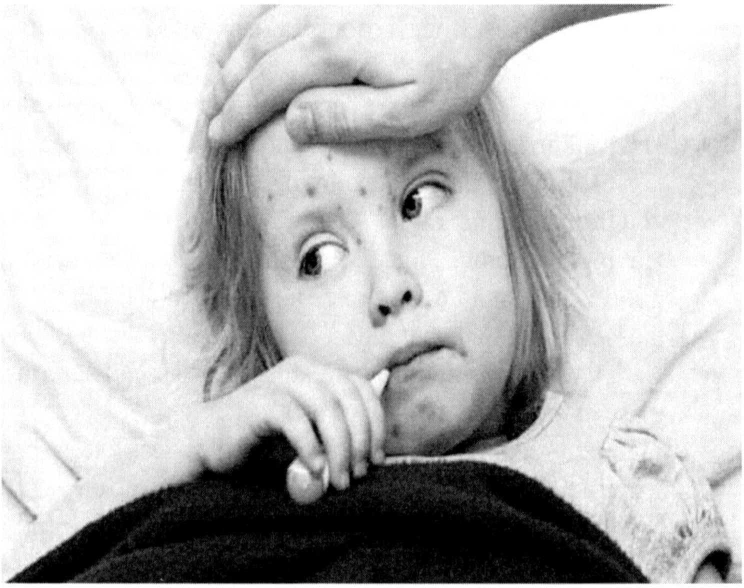

66. Measles

An infectious viral disease, measles has become very common in the present times. The infection leads to the emergence of rashes, which first appear on the cheeks and then spread over to the trunks, palms and soles. Initially pink in color, the rashes grow darker as time passes. Measles may also be accompanied with fever, diarrhea and watering of the eyes. They might result from personal contact, droplets from coughs and sneezes, immunodeficiency due to HIV/AIDS, malnutrition or vitamin A deficiency and usually last for about 5 days. In the following lines, we have listed the home remedies for measles.

Home Remedy for Measles

- Lemon juice is known to be beneficial for treating measles. Take 15ml - 25 ml of lemon juice, diluted with water.
- Mix ½ tsp each of licorice and honey and consume on a daily basis. This is beneficial for a person suffering from measles.

- Powder dried turmeric roots. Take about ½ tsp of this powder, with honey and juice of a few bitter gourd leaves. This is a good way to cure a person suffering from measles.
- Have lukewarm water for baths and if possible, add neem leaves to the bathing water. It will be helpful in relieving you from the itching.
- Having fresh orange juice, when struck with measles, is a good way to get healthy once again. Intake about two glasses of the juice per day.
- Barley water is beneficial in treating measles. Consume a glass of this on an everyday basis.
- Eggplant seeds are effective in curing measles. Take ½ to 1 gram of these seeds everyday, for about three days.]
- Mix equal amounts of tamarind seeds and turmeric and grind it well. Have this mixture, in a dose of 350 to 400 grams, three times a day.
- Having a balanced diet is essential in treating measles. Avoid having milk products, spicy food and junk foods.

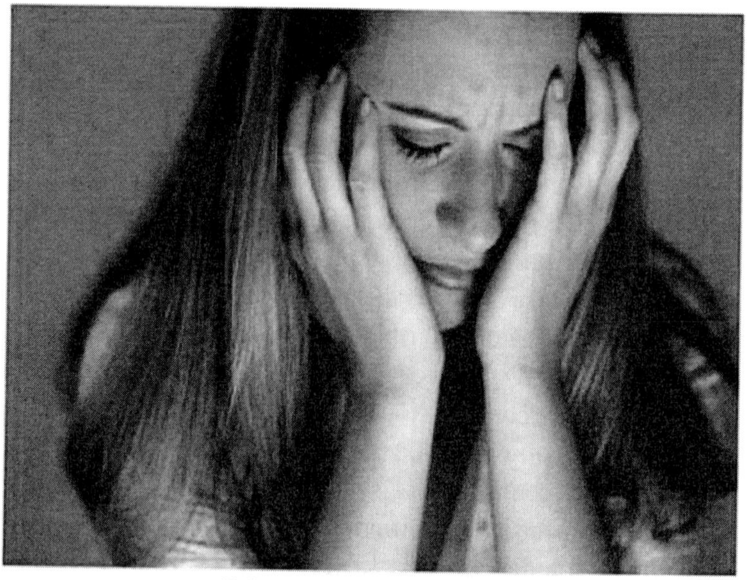

67. Menopausal Disorder

Menopause marks the period when there is a permanent cessation of menstruation. It occurs in women when they are in their mid-forties to mid-fifties. It is a significant period for a woman, as it marks the end of her reproductive stage. Most women suffer from menopausal disorder at this stage. During menopause, the most affected regions of the body are the endocrine glands, gonads, thyroid and pituitary glands. Some of the symptoms seen in women going through menopause are hot flushes, night sweats, tension, irritability, headache, palpitation, insomnia, numbness, depression, dizziness and lack interest in sex. Though menopausal disorder is a natural phenomenon, its symptoms can be alleviated, using the home remedies listed below.

Home Remedy for Menopausal Disorder

- Beet juice is very beneficial for the women going through menopause. Extract the juice of beetroot and have it in small quantities, usually 60 to 90 ml, at a time. Drink this juice three times in a day.

- Soak one tsp carrot seeds in a glass of cow's milk for about ten minutes. Strain the milk and throw away the seeds. Consume this milk once in a day.
- Liquorice is an effective home remedy to alleviate menopausal problems. Consume a tsp of powdered liquorice on a daily basis.
- Indian spikenard is valuable in treating menopausal tension. It is advisable to have it a dose of 2 grams per day.
- Increase the consumption of vitamin D. Some of the foods rich in vitamin D are beef, bread, cheese, eggs, milk and breakfast cereal.
- The diet for a female suffering from menopausal disorder must include fruits, nuts, vegetables, sprouted seeds, alfalfa, soybeans, cabbage and olive oil. All of them provide relief from menopausal problems.
- Exercising regularly reduces the symptoms of menopausal disorder, solving the problem to quite an extent.

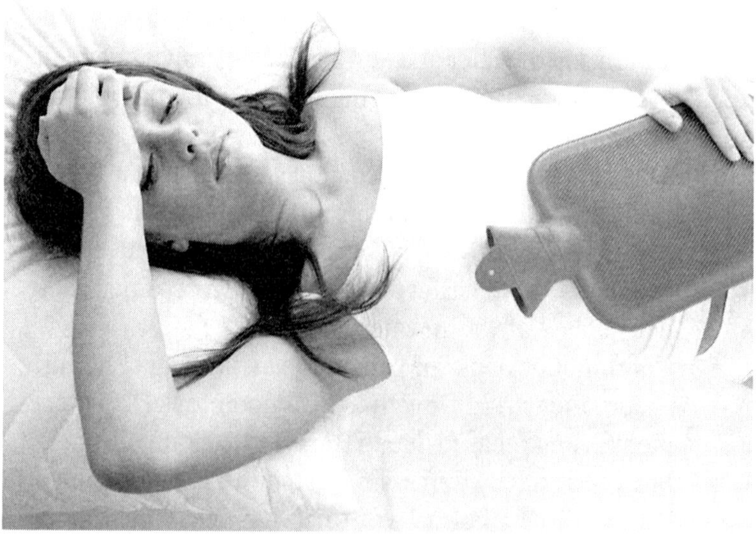

68. Menstrual Problems

Menstruation is the monthly flow of blood from a woman's body. It is nothing, but the shedding of the uterus lining, which helps in cleansing the inner surface of the womb. Menstrual flow is related with the function of ovulation or reproduction. A natural phenomenon, it occurs regularly in females, throughout their reproductive age. During menstruation, or periods as it is more commonly known as, females face problems such as menorrhagia or excessive menstrual flow, amenorrhea or stoppage of menstrual flow, dysmenorrhoea or painful menstruation, premenstrual tension and menstrual cramps. To curb all these problems, the best way would be to retort to the home remedies, some of which have been mentioned below.

Home Remedy for Menstrual Problems

- The best way to treat menstrual problems would be to have parsley juice, in combination with any other juice.

You can mix 75 ml of parsley with beet, carrot or cucumber juice, of the same quantity.

- Take a cup of water and add a piece of fresh ginger to it. Make sure to pound the ginger before you put it in the water. Boil the water for a few minutes and then, strain it. Mix a little sugar to the decoction and consume it, after it cools down a bit. Repeat this three times in a day.
- Sesame seeds prove to be beneficial in case of menstrual problems. Take half a tsp of powdered sesame seeds, with a glass of warm water, two times a day.
- Consumption of unripe papaya is beneficial for securing a proper menstrual flow. It is also good for girls whose menses have ceased due to stress or tension.
- Prepare a bath by immersing an entire Chickpea plant in hot water. This is helpful when there is immense pain during menstruation.
- The herb of Marigold is helpful in reducing the pain during menstruation and also increasing the flow. It is advisable to have a tablespoon of this, two times a day.
- For women who face the problem of excessive menstruation, banana flower would provide an effective remedy. Boil a banana flower in some water, until it turns soft. Take it out, crush it and have it with a cup of curd.
- In half liter of water, put 6 grams of coriander seeds and boil it until only half the quantity remains. Sweeten the decoction, with sugar or honey, and have it when warm.
- Extract the juice of fresh mango bark. Mix 10 ml of the juice with 120 ml of water. Have this mixture in a dose of 1 or 2 tsp, every one hour.
- You can also consume the juice of fresh mango bark, after adding an egg white or some mucilage and a small quantity of the kernel of a poppy, to it.

- Boil 90 gm of the bark of Ashoka tree, in 30 ml of milk and 360 ml of water. Keep on boiling until the total quantity is reduced to about 90 ml. Drink this in 2 or 3 doses. Start consuming this decoction from the fourth day of the monthly period, until the bleeding is checked.
- Consume thirteen to twenty-five grams of the Indian barbery herb, during excessive bleeding.
- Prepare an infusion of the herb 'rough chaff' by steeping 15 gm of it, in 250 ml of boiling water. Strain the mixture and drink when warm.
- Boil two tablespoons of hermal seeds in half a liter of water. Once the decoction is reduced to 1/3rd its quantity, stop boiling. Strain it and let it cool down a bit. Have it in a dose of 15 to 30 ml, per day.
- Take half a liter of water and boil it with five large heads of hemps, until it reduces to one-half. Strain the decoction, cool it down and have it before going to bed.

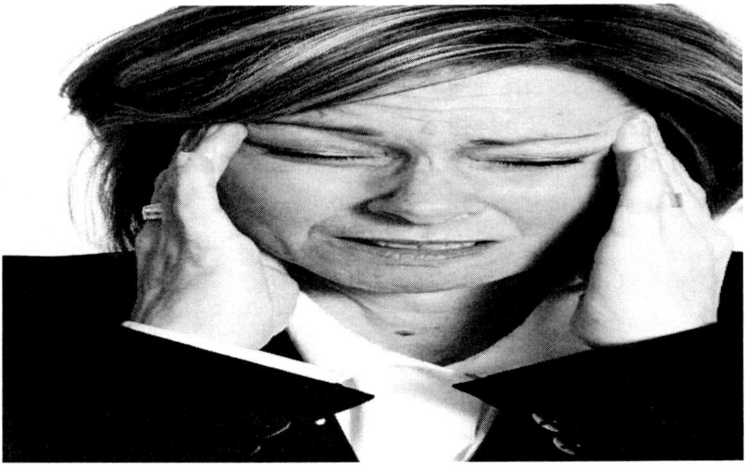

69. Migraine

Migraine is the name given to severe headaches, normally lasting from 4 to 72 hours. It is mainly felt s pulsing or throbbing in one area of the head. During migraine, there is contraction or dilation of the blood vessels. Some of the factors that can trigger a migraine attack anxiety, stress, lack of food or sleep, exposure to light and hormonal changes (in women). In women, menstruation can also result in migraine. The symptoms of migraine are pain on one side of the head, a short period of depression, irritability and loss of appetite, pounding pain, nausea and vomiting as well as numbness or weakness in an arm or leg or on one side of the face. This severe headache can, however, be cured, naturally using home remedies.

Home Remedy for Migraine

- Migraine can be treated effectively with the help of fresh grape juice. Grind grapes to extract the juice. Consume the juice in the concentrated form, without adding water.
- Increase the intake of niacin (vitamin B3), as it has been found to be helpful in alleviating migraine pain. Some of the foods rich in niacin are yeast, whole wheat, green leafy vegetables, tomatoes, nuts, sunflower seeds, liver and fish.

- Cabbage leaves are helpful in relieving the pain of a migraine headache. Squash cabbage leaves and place them in a cloth. Place the cloth on your forehead for sometime. Once the cabbage leaves become dry, remove the cloth and make a fresh one.
- Lemon peel is helpful in solving migraine headache. Grind lemon peel to form a paste and apply it on the forehead. Let it dry and then rinse off with cool water.
- A mixture of carrot juice, either with spinach, beet or cucumber juice, works effectively in curing migraine. Combine 300 ml of carrot juice with 200 ml of any other juice and drink it.
- You can also mix 100 ml each of beet and cucumber juices, with 300 ml of carrot juice and drink it on a regular basis.
- Massaging the forehead with primrose oil is beneficial in curing migraine. It works as an excellent anti-inflammatory agent, preventing any kind of constriction in the blood vessels.
- Include garlic in your diet. Either chew a piece of garlic in the raw form or mix it with other food items.
- Another effective method would be to have chamomile tea. This is effective in reducing the occurrence of migraine.
- Taking lukewarm water enema is effective. It cleanses the bowels, thereby removing the toxins from the body and helping prevent migraine.
- Take some sandalwood powder and add a few drops of water to it, so as to form a paste. Apply this paste on the forehead and let it dry. Once dry, rub it off by hand and wash it.
- It is advisable to avoid direct sunlight; smoking and drinking alcohol, as all these can aggravate migraine.

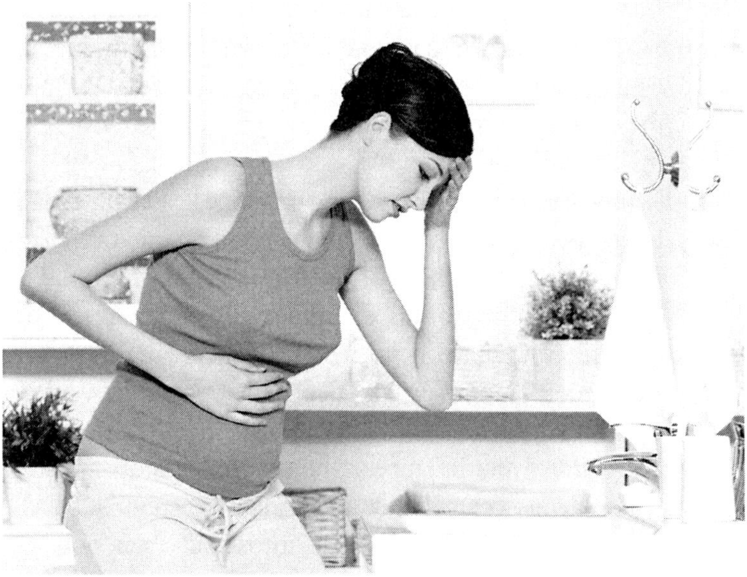

70. Morning Sickness

The feeling of nausea, which might result in vomiting, experienced during the period of pregnancy is called morning sickness. Almost 50 to 80 percent of the pregnant women face this problem during the first trimester of pregnancy. However, in some women, it can last till the third trimester as well. Though it can occur at any time of the day, morning sickness is usually more prevalent in the morning hours. Some of the main causes of morning sickness are chemical changes in the body, hormonal changes or hormonal imbalance, sensitive gastrointestinal tract, vitamin B deficiency and strong odors. The best way to deal with morning sickness would be to resort to the natural ways.

Home Remedy for Morning Sickness

- The best way to deal with morning sickness would be to have a cup of ginger tea, early in the morning.
- Mix a tablespoon each of apple cider vinegar and honey, in a glass of cool water. It is an effective way to cure morning sickness.

- It is advisable to have 6 small meals in a day, instead of 3 large ones. This might reduce the effect of morning sickness.
- Mix a teaspoon of limejuice, mint juice and sugar. Have this decoction three times a day. It is a good way to deal with morning sickness.
- Avoid having fried items as well as fatty and spicy foods.
- Take some wheat germ and dissolve it in warm milk. Have it every hour. This will prove to be effective in curing morning sickness.
- Consume a high protein snack before going to bed. This is a good way to resolve morning sickness.
- Extract the juice of 20 to 25 curry leaves. Thereafter, add 2 tsp of fresh limejuice and 1 tsp of honey to it. Intake this mixture 3-4 times in a day.
- Mix 1/2 tsp ginger juice, 1 tsp fresh limejuice, 1 tsp mint juice and 1 tsp honey. Have this mixture 3-4 times a day.
- Put 3 drops of lavender oil and 1 drop of peppermint in a humidifier. This would emit a good fragrance in the room, which would be effective in treating morning sickness.
- Vitamin B deficiency can also cause morning sickness. In such a case, it is advisable to include salads, wheat, vegetables, bananas, sea food and chicken in your diet.
- Have food items that are rich in calcium, protein and complex carbohydrates.
- Having a glass of lemon juice, first thing in the morning, is also beneficial in treating morning sickness.
- Drink lots of fluids. Consuming large quantities of water and fresh juice will keep the body temperature under control and reduce the chances of nausea or vomiting.

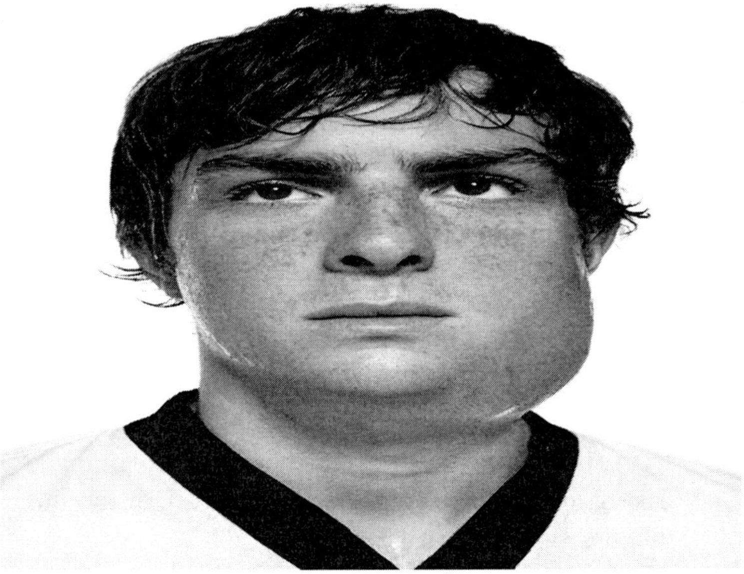

71. Mumps

A highly contagious disease, mumps is an infection caused mostly in the salivary glands and gonads. At times, it might be seen at the other parts of the body as well. People usually experience mumps in the age group of 5 to 15 years. The main symptom of mumps comprises of the swelling in the salivary glands. Mostly, a person is infected with mumps only once in a lifetime. However, there might be rare cases, where the infection occurs for the second time as well. Though there are no specific treatments for mumps, they can be alleviated with the help of home remedies, some of which have been mentioned below.

Home Remedy for Mumps

- Rub Chebulic myroblan herb in water. Apply this paste over the swelling. This is an effective home remedy for curing mumps.

- Smear the leaves of peepal leaves with clarified butter and warm them over fire. Place these leaves over the swelled area and bandage it properly.
- Peel one side of the herb Indian aloe. Warm the peeled side and sprinkle some turmeric powder over it, along with the extract of Indian barbery. Place it over the inflamed area and bandage it properly.
- The seeds of asparagus and fenugreek are beneficial in treating mumps. Take equal proportions of asparagus and fenugreek seeds and grind them. Adding some water, make a paste out of it. Apply this paste over the swellings to get relief.
- Grind dry ginger and make a paste with water. Apply this paste over the infected area. Not only would this reduce the swelling, but also subsidize the pain.
- Mash the leaves of margosa and add some turmeric powder and water, to form a paste. Apply this paste over the affected area. It would prove effective in treating mumps.
- It is advisable to avoid any kind of acidic food. The patient suffering from mumps should not be given citrus juices and curd. Instead, water and vegetable soup should be preferred.
- Liquids like rice water, flavored with some ghee and taken along with raw mango pickle, are amongst the ideal foods during mumps.

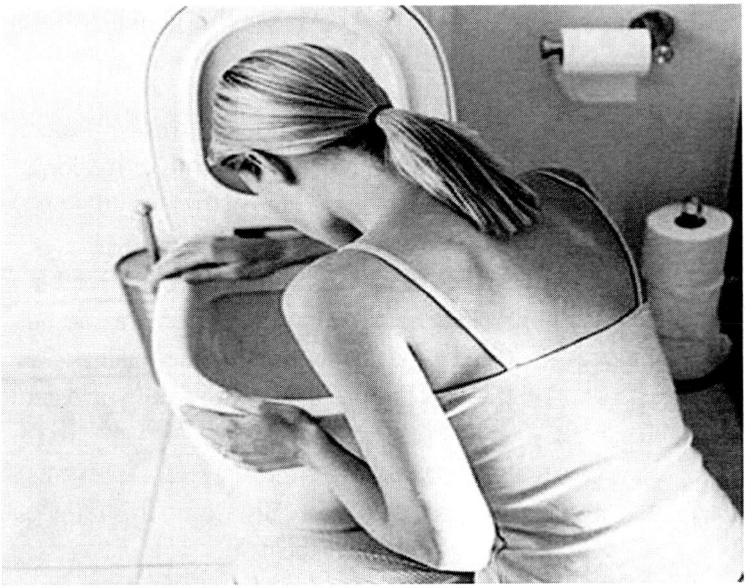

72. Nausea

Nausea can be described as a sensation of unease and discomfort in the stomach, with an urge to vomit. It is not a sickness in itself, rather a symptom, which might be experienced in case of numerous diseases or disorders. Nausea can be seen in case of indigestion, morning sickness, motion and sea sickness, stress, chemotherapy, consumption of drugs and alcohol, overeating, food intolerance and different illnesses. The main symptoms of the nauseating feeling are an urge to puke, stomach pain, dizziness and sweating. The condition is not very grave and can be treated at home only.

Home Remedy for Nausea

- The best way to treat nausea, at home, would be to have a cup of ginger tea.
- Mix 1 tbsp each of apple cider vinegar and honey in a glass of cold water. Have this mixture when you feel nauseous.

- In 2 cups of water, boil ½ cup of rice for about 10minutes. Once cooked, strain the rice water and have it when warm.
- Mix a few tsp of wheat germ in warm milk. Have this mixture every one hour. This is helpful in treating nausea.
- Consuming 1/2 tsp grounded cumin seed, along with water, is beneficial in treating nausea.
- Having fiber rich food proves to be helpful when a person is suffering from nausea. Some of the foods rich in fiber are banana, rice, apple sauce and brown bread.
- It is advisable to have a healthy diet. Include fruits and vegetables in your diet and exclude oily, spicy as well as fried foods.
- Have peppermint or chamomile tea. This would be helpful in treating the nauseating feeling.
- Put ½ tsp baking soda in a glass of lukewarm water and consume it. However, avoid it during pregnancy.
- Sip a glass of water that has a fresh lime squeezed in it. You can also add a pinch of salt to it.

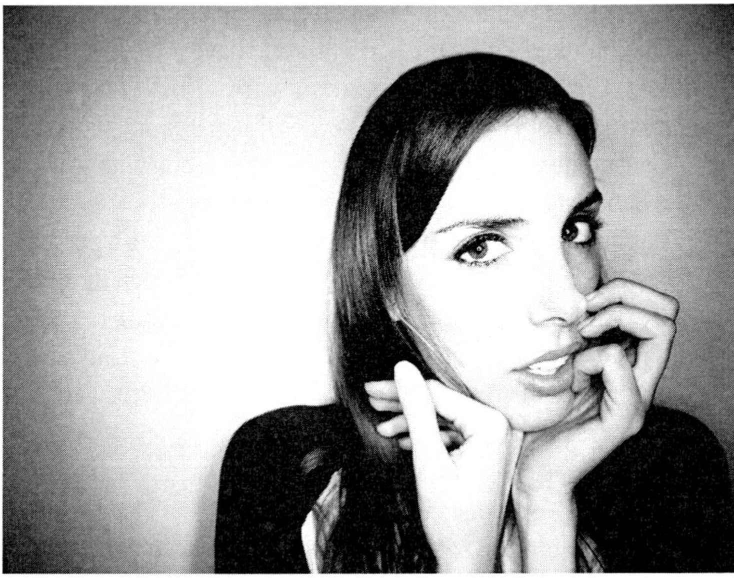

73. Nervousness

Nervousness is a feeling of restlessness, apprehension and worry that a person goes through when he faces a stressful situation. The most common symptoms of nervousness are palpitations, muscle tension, dry mouth, sweating, lack of concentration, sleeplessness, gasping (a.k.a. hyper ventilation), sick feeling in the stomach and a strong anticipation of something disastrous ahead. The best way to deal with the problem would be to realize the cause of anxiety and take preventive action. At the same time, there are certain home remedies that can work beneficially in removing nervousness.

Home Remedy for Nervousness

- Inhale the fragrance while peeling an orange. Alternatively, drop an orange in a pot of boiling water and inhale the vapor.
- You can also add 2 tablespoons honey and 1 teaspoon nutmeg in a cup of orange juice and drink the mixture.

- Apply rosemary oil on your forehead. You can also put dried rosemary herb in the boiling-hot water and let it steep for 15 minutes. Drain the decoction and sip it when a bit cool.
- Grate two onions add 2 cups celery to it. Use this mixture in food or salad. It would help to relieve the restlessness.
- Fill the bath tub with lukewarm water. Add 1/3 cup each of baking soda and ginger and enjoy a warm bath.
- Soak 8 to 10 raw almonds in water overnight. Peel them in the morning and add enough water to form a paste. Now, add one tsp nutmeg, with a pinch of ginger in it. Consume this paste at bedtime.
- For people suffering from shaking hands and finger control problem, two cups of tea each day, with one tablespoon of honey in each cup, would prove beneficial.
- The most simple of all remedies would be to place a drop of primrose oil on the tongue.
- Drinking catnip, chamomile, hops, horsetail, marshmallow, peach leaf, peppermint and spearmint tea has been found to be useful in curing nervousness.

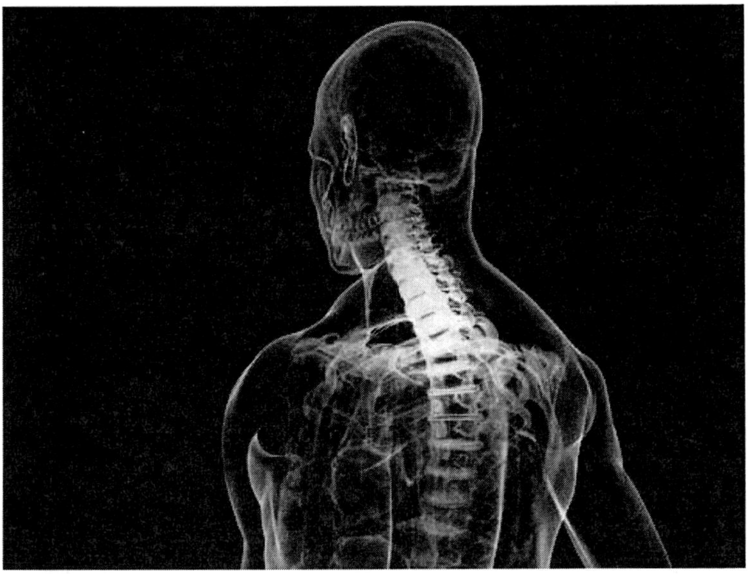

74. Neuritis

An inflammation or swelling of a single nerve or nerves is termed as neuritis. If, at a time, different groups of nerves, in various parts of the body, get inflamed, the condition is called polyneuritis. The causes of neuritis include presence of toxins due to faulty living habits and nutrition as well as injury or pressure over a nerve trunk. Neuritis is mainly associated with a tingling or burning sensation and pain in the affected area. Other symptoms include numbness, loss of sensation, and paralysis of the nearby muscles. Neuritis can be treated using some home remedies.

Home Remedy for Neuritis

- Soya bean milk is beneficial in treating neuritis. Add a tsp of honey in a cup of soy milk and consume it every night, before going to bed.
- Boil 1/4 cup pearled barley grain in half a cup of water. Once the concoction gets reduced to 1/4th, strain it. For a better

effect, mix it with half a glass of buttermilk and the juice of half a lime.

- Carrots and spinach are effective in treating neuritis. Combine 300 ml of carrot juice and 200 ml of spinach juice. Have this combination regularly.
- The flowers of orange are beneficial in curing neuritis. Eat fresh orange flowers, along with honey. Another method would be to distill water from the flowers and drink it on a daily basis.
- Increase your intake of vitamin D.
- Soak soya beans in water for about 12 hours. Thereafter, peel them and grind to make a paste. Add some water to the paste and place it on fire, until the first boil comes. Strain the mixture and have it when warm.

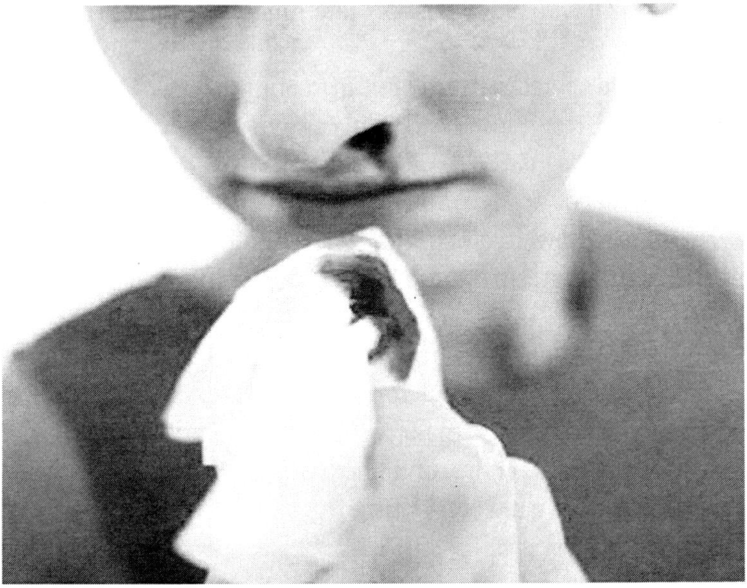

75. Nose Bleed

Nose bleeding is a common ailment that is found in children and adults alike. It is mainly the result of the vulnerability of the nose lining that contains various tiny blood vessels, which tend to bleed easily. There are various reasons or causes of nose bleeding, such as injury to the nose, infection of the mucous membrane, dryness, cold, nose picking and also a sudden impact or blow to the nose. Still, there may be instances where nosebleed occurs without any specific cause. Most of the nose bleeding occurs in the front part of the nose and can be stopped easily. In case the bleeding takes place internally, you need to consult a doctor.

Home Remedy for Nose Bleed

- The best way to stop bleeding in the nose would be to blow the nose, forcefully, once. By doing this, the clot, if any, will come out. Once the clot is out, the opening in the nose will contract itself.

- Put a drop or two of lemon juice in the nostril that is bleeding. This is an effective way to stop nose bleed.
- Saline water serves as a good natural remedy for treating nose bleed. For this, put a pinch of salt in half a glass of water and spray it inside the nose.
- Dip a cotton ball in apple cider vinegar and apply it on the bleeding nose. It helps the blood to congeal and will bring the bleeding to a stop.
- When nosebleed occurs, you need to make sure that the surroundings are not dry. Humidify the air with a good air humidifier. This would prevent the nose from working exceedingly hard, thereby preventing bleeding.
- In a pint of water, add a tsp of goldenseal. Put the solution in a pan and place it on flame. Once the first boil comes, turn off the flame and let the decoction settle down. When it gets cool, snuff some into the nostrils. Repeat this a few times a day. Apply an ice pack on the exterior of the nose. This is an easy and effective way to cure nose bleeding.
- Placing a wet towel on the head has been found to be beneficial in curing nose bleeding.

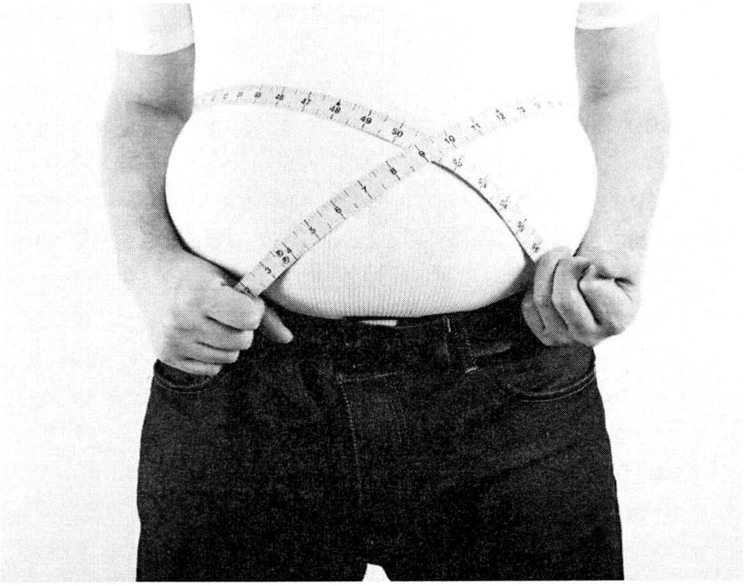

76. Obesity

Obesity is the condition where a person has excessive deposit or storage of fat in his/her body. It can affect a person in any and every age group and is also not restricted by sex. Obesity is found more in people who consume food in large quantities and lead a sedentary live. A serious health hazard, the extra fat puts strain on the heart, kidneys, liver and joints of hips, knees and ankles. The causes of obesity include overeating, low basal metabolism, thyroid or pituitary gland disorders, sedentary lifestyle, genetic factors and hormonal imbalance. While being overweight refers to an increase in overall body weight, including essential body tissues, obesity refers only to excessive fat tissues. However, obesity can be treated effectively at home, resorting to some natural ways.

Home Remedies for Obesity

- The easiest and effective remedy to fight obesity would be to have 10 grams of honey, along with a glass of warm water. Consume this in the morning, on an empty stomach. If found effective, the dose can be increased with time.

- You can also mix juice of half a lime and one teaspoon of fresh honey in a glass of lukewarm water. Have this early in the morning, followed by every few hours intake.
- Consuming 10-12 fully grown curry leaves every morning, for 3 months, is found beneficial in dealing with the problem of obesity.
- Have one or two tomatoes, on an empty stomach, every morning. This has been found to be effective in curing obesity.
- In a glass of boiling water, add ginger and lemon slices. Steep for sometime and strain the water. Have this decoction when warm. Not only would it treat obesity, it would also control overeating tendency.
- In a cup of water, add 3 tsp limejuice, ¼ tsp powdered black pepper and 1 tsp honey. Have this concoction regularly, once a day, for 3 months.
- Soak a handful of jujube or Indian plum leaves overnight. Strain the water in the morning and consume on an empty stomach. It will prove beneficial in curing obesity.
- Include loads of cabbage in your diet. You can have its leaves raw or boiled. You can also make a vegetable out of it or use it in salads.
- Take out fresh carrot juice, add a little water and churn it in a blender. Filter the juice and drink it.
- Include French beans, jackfruits, grapes, figs, peaches, phalsa and guava in the diet.
- Having green tea has been found to be beneficial in treating obesity. You can also consume tea made from dandelion root.
- In a cup of lukewarm water, add ½ tbsp honey and ½ tsp holy basil paste. Consume this everyday, for treating obesity.

- Horse gram can help cure obesity. Soak 1-2 tbsp horse gram in a glass of water and keep it overnight. Filter the concoction the next morning and have it on an empty stomach.
- Make ginger paste and add a small amount to honey to it. Consume this along with ½ tsp natural guggul. It will prove effective in treating obesity.

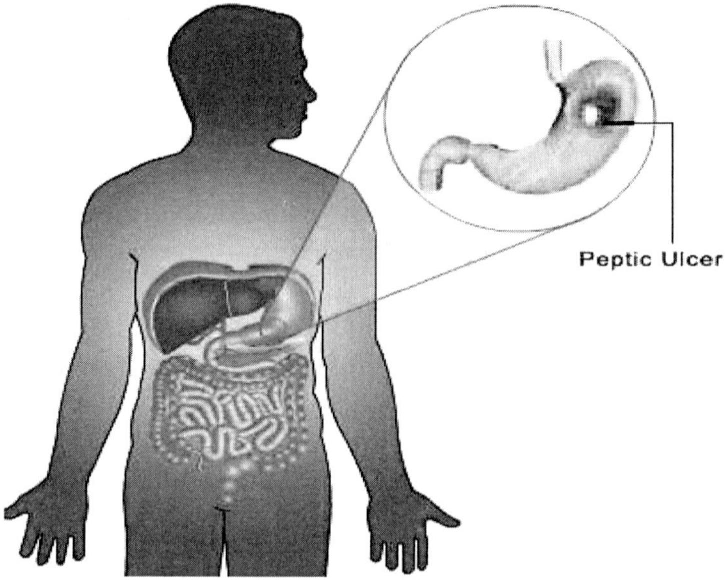

77. Peptic Ulcer

The erosion caused in the inner lining of the stomach and intestinal tract has been given the name of 'peptic ulcer'. While the ulcer in stomach is known as gastric ulcer, the one in intestinal tract, or duodenum, is called duodenal ulcer. When gastric ulcer and duodenal ulcer are clubbed together, they are known as peptic ulcer. The main causes of peptic ulcers are hyperacidity, excessive intake of alcohol, overeating, high intake of spicy foods, food poisoning, high intake of coffee, smoking and presence of helicobacter pylori. The symptoms of peptic ulcer include sharp and severe pain, along with discomfort, in the upper part of the abdomen. When a peptic ulcer develops, the stomach swells due to excessive flatulence, mental tension, insomnia and gradual weakening of the body. Peptic ulcer, however, can be treated at home using some natural remedies.

Home Remedy for Peptic Ulcer

- The most effective home remedy for treating peptic ulcer is to eat bananas everyday. It is an excellent way to neutralize the hyperacidity of the gastric juices. Banana milk shake is also beneficial in curing peptic ulcer.
- Having cold milk, without sugar, is effective in reducing the acid, thereby providing relief from burning sensation one encounters in peptic ulcer.
- Prepare a paste of 10 grams drumsticks leaves and water. Mix this paste in half a cup of yoghurt. Have this mixture everyday, to cure peptic ulcer.
- In 250 ml of water, soak 15 grams leaves of wood apple and keep it overnight. Strain this concoction in the morning and have it.
- Applying a hot pack over the abdomen region is one of the effective ways of curing peptic ulcer.
- Cabbage and carrot, when mixed as juices, have been found to be beneficial in treating peptic ulcer. In half a liter of water, boil 250 grams cabbage until it is reduced to half. In a similar way, prepare carrot juice. Now, combine 125 ml of each juice. Once cool, drink it two times in a day.
- Tea made from fenugreek seeds is effective in curing peptic ulcer. When coated with water, fenugreek seeds become slightly mucilaginous, which helps in treating the ulcer.
- Combining carrot juice with spinach (or beet) and cucumber is effective in treating peptic ulcer. You can either mix 300ml carrot juice and 200 ml spinach juice or combine 300 ml carrot juice and 100 ml each of beet and cucumber juice, to make 500 ml of juice. Consume this daily.
- Blanch 5 almonds everyday and extract their milk. Drink this milk everyday, as it provides protein and also binds the acid in stomach.

- Drinking raw goat milk is effective in peptic ulcers treatment. For best results, drink this juice three times a day.
- Lime is beneficial in curing peptic ulcer. The citric acid and mineral salts present in it help treat the ulcer. You can either have lime juice or use it in salads.

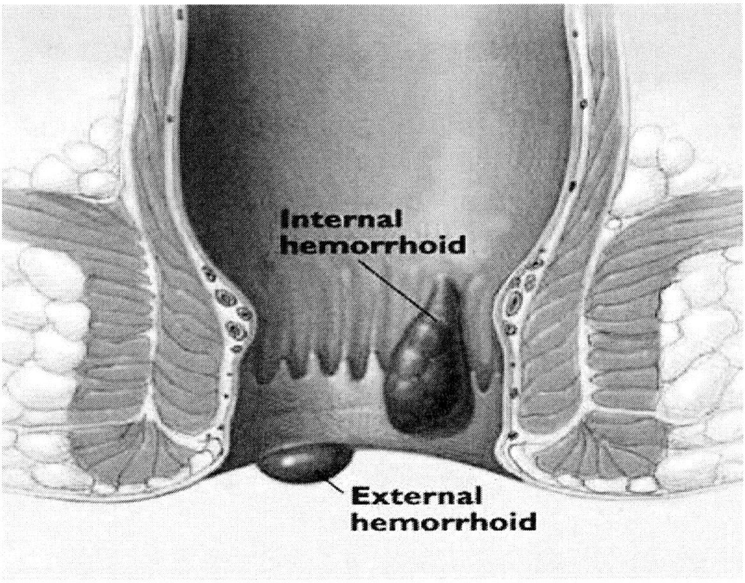

78. Piles

Hemorrhoids, more popularly known as piles, can be described as a condition where the veins around the anus or lower rectum swell or get inflamed. It is due to this that a person faces difficulty in passing stool. Piles can be dry as well as bleeding. Even dry piles can result in bleeding, if they continue for a long time. There are two types of piles - internal piles, not seen but felt, and external piles, visible around the exterior of the anus region. Increased pressure from the internal or external veins can be one of the reasons of piles. Some other causes include low fiber diet, pregnancy, aging, hereditary factors, chronic constipation and anal intercourse. Piles can be treated using some home remedies as well.

Home Remedy for Piles

- The best way to treat piles at home would be to have a mixture of yoghurt and black mustard. In a bowl of yoghurt, mix some powdered black mustard. While having it, make sure to chew the mustard very carefully. After this, drink a glass of buttermilk.

- In a bowl of water, soak peels of a pomegranate. Place the bowl on flame and let this water boil. Turn off the flame, strain the concoction and let it cool down. Drink this once in the morning and once in the evening.
- Prepare some buttermilk, using cow's milk. Add peppercorns, ginger and rock salt to this. Have this mixture two times a day.
- Put 10 gm black mustard in 150 ml goat's milk. In this, add 5 gm sugar. Drink this mixture in the morning, everyday.
- In a bowl of yoghurt, put a few flowers of tamarind plant and some pomegranate juice. Once you have blended this well, add coriander and ginger pastes to it. Consume this after lunch. It will help pacify the pain.
- Grind some dry slices of yam into a powder. In 160 grams of this powder, add 80 grams white leadwort. Now, add 10 grams black pepper and 500 grams of jaggery. Mix well and make small tablets or capsules of this mixture. Have one piece each in the morning and evening.
- For bleeding piles, keep 1/4 liter goat's milk for curdling overnight. In the morning, add an equal amount of carrot juice and blend it. Drink this mixture. Alternatively, freshly prepared goat's milk yogurt, consumed with freshly chopped carrots, is also beneficial in treating piles.
- Radish is effective in curing piles. Extract the juice of white radish and mix it with honey. Apply this mixture on the affected region. This will prove helpful in treating piles.
- For instant relief, applying coconut oil on the affected region will be your best bet.
- Extract the seeds of ripe mangoes and dry them in the sun. Once dry, grind them into a fine powder. Store this

powder in bottles. Consuming 2 gm of this powder, with honey, twice a day will be effective in curing piles.

- Mix ½ tsp each of ginger juice, lime juice and mint leaves juice, in 1 tbsp honey. Have this mixture once a day. It will be helpful in treating piles.
- Take 1 tbsp each of roasted black cumin seeds and cumin seeds (not roasted). Mix this well and add to a glass of cold water. Drink this concoction once every day.
- In a cup of milk, mash a ripe banana. Have this mixture 3 to 4 times in a day, to stop the pain experienced during piles.
- Soak 3 to 4 figs in a glass of water and keep them overnight. Have them early in the morning, on an empty stomach.
- Extract the juice of bitter gourd leaves. Mix 2 tsp of this juice in a glass of buttermilk and have it on an empty stomach, every morning.
- Extract about 150 ml of turnip juice. Consume this juice after combining it with any other vegetable juice, such as spinach, watercress or carrots.

79. Pneumonia

Pneumonia, an infectious disease, causes inflammation of the lungs. One of the most dangerous diseases, pneumonia is threatening if both the lungs of the ailing person get affected. This condition is termed as double pneumonia. Some of the causes of pneumonia are bronchiectasis, excessive smoking, chronic alcohol misuse, intravenous drug misuse, weakened immune system, cystic fibrosis and lung cancer. The real cause of pneumonia is the weakened immune system of the body, a result of the toxins present in the air passages and lungs. Chest pain, fever, chills, leucocytosis, cough, labored breathing, fatigue, anorexia, headache and bloody sputum are some of the symptoms of pneumonia. However, pneumonia can be treated using home remedies.

Home Remedy for Pneumonia

- In the early stages of pneumonia, the best treatment would be to have tea prepared from fenugreek seeds. Have four cups of this tea everyday. Along with this, no other nourishment or food should be taken. You can reduce the quantity of intake once the condition improves.
- Garlic acts favorably in curing pneumonia. It can be added to the food prepared for the patient. Alternatively, garlic paste can also be applied over the chest. Apart from

bringing down the body temperature, it tones down respiration and pulse.

- Steep 15 gm sesame seeds in 250 ml water. Mix this infusion with 1 tablespoon each of honey and linseed. Also add a pinch of table salt and consume. This is very effective in treating pneumonia.
- Carrot juice, when combined with beet and cucumber juices or spinach juice, is also beneficial in curing pneumonia. In 300 ml carrot juice, mix in either 200 ml of spinach juice or 100 ml each of beet and cucumber juice.
- Another effective home remedy would be to rub some turpentine oil over the patient's rib cage. After this, cover the area with a warm cloth.
- Extract juice of 5 to 6 Holy Basil leaves. To this, add some black pepper. Consume this after every 6 hours.

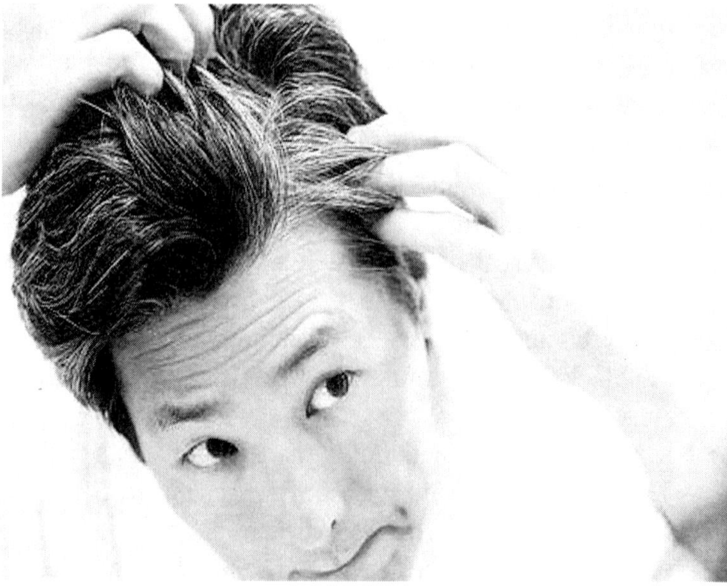

80. Premature Graying of Hair

Premature graying of hair is a normal occurrence in people these days. It is characterized by fading out of hair, with the color draining from it. The condition can affect anyone, causing a young person to look much older than he/she actually is. The actual cause of premature graying is lack of oil gland production in the follicles of the scalp. In such a condition, hair looses the nutrition that it needs and starts turning gray. Diet also plays an important role in premature graying of the hair. Especially the deficiency of Vitamin B, copper, iron and iodine causes premature graying. At times, it also results from excessive worry and anxiety. However, the dullness of the hair can be removed easily, regaining the shine and radiance, by resorting to some natural remedies.

Home Remedy for Premature Graying of Hair

- One of the best home remedies for premature graying of hair comprises of curry leaves. Include them in your daily diet. Alternatively, you can put some curry leaves in coconut oil and boil it. Strain the oil and let it cool down. Apply it over the scalp.

- Dry a few pieces of ribbed gourd in the sun. Soak them in coconut oil for about 3 to 4 hours. After this, boil it until the residue becomes black and cool it down a bit. Massage the scalp with the residue.
- Extract juice from fresh leaves of amaranth vegetable. Apply this juice on the hair. It will prove helpful in retaining the black color of hair and also aid the growth of new hair.
- Massage the scalp with butter made out of cow's milk. This should be applied at least two times in a week.
- Indian gooseberry is beneficial in treating premature graying of hair. Cut the fruit into pieces and dry them. Once dried, put them in coconut oil, until the solid matter becomes dusty or powdered. Apply on the hair.
- Mix a tsp of Indian gooseberry juice with a tsp of almond oil and few drops of lime juice. Apply this mixture on your hair and keep it overnight. In the morning, wash the hair. This is an effective home remedy for treating premature graying of hair.
- Avoid having refined flour and sugar, soft drinks, pastries, jam, too spicy food, hot food, chilies and oily food.
- Eat a lot of fresh fruits and vegetables. They are effective in treating premature graying of hair.
- Mix a liter of yoghurt with a tablespoon of yeast. Have a bowl of this mixture before every meal, as it is effective in treating premature graying.

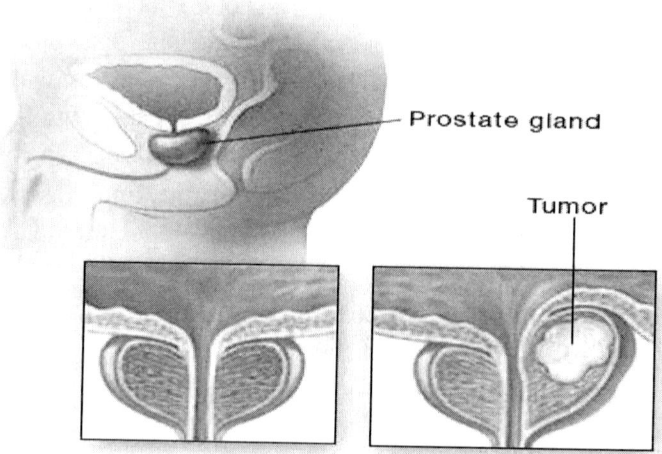

81. Prostate Disorders

Prostate disorder is a common ailment that can affect men of all ages. Prostate is a gland that is similar, in shape and size, to a chestnut. Situated at the base of the urinary bladder, encircling the urethra, this gland might swell, at times, blocking urine output. This leads to prostate disorder, which in turn causes pain, urination problems and sexual problems. The pain might extend to the lower back and in the hips, legs and feet as well. Prostrate disorder also increases the risk of infection and cancer. One of the main symptoms of prostrate disorder is that though a person feels like urinating, nothing actually happens. This can, however, be resolved by resorting to some home remedies.

Home Remedy for Prostate Disorders

- Holy basil is very effective in treating prostrate disorder. In summers, you can mix 1 tsp of holy basil juice with a tsp of yoghurt and consume it once in a day. In winters, mix 1 tsp of the juice with a tsp of honey.

- An easy, yet effective way to treat prostrate would be to sit in a warm water tub for half an hour. This would help in reducing the swelling and also provide relief against pain.
- Another easy remedy is to increase the intake of water. This would be an effective way to cure prostrate disorder.
- Include a lot of vegetables, fruits, nuts and seeds in your diet. Avoid having starchy, sweet, spicy and seasoned foods. Alcoholic and caffeinated beverages should also be completely avoided.
- Pumpkin seeds act beneficially in treating prostrate disorder. 50 grams of the seeds needs to taken every day, either in cooked food or in powdered form.
- Mix 200 ml of spinach juice and 300 ml of carrot juice. Consume this mixture every morning.

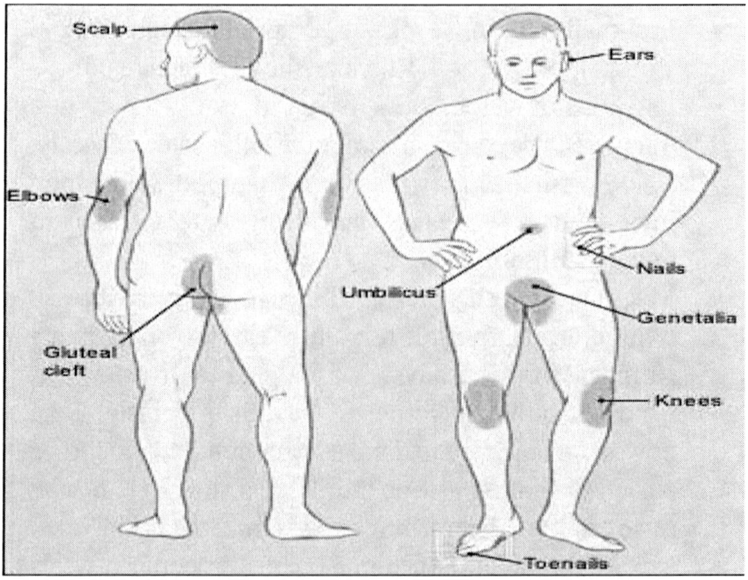

82. Psoriasis

A chronic skin disease, psoriasis is basically of five types - plague psoriasis, guttate psoriasis, pustular psoriasis, inverse psoriasis and erythrodermic psoriasis. It is characterized by thick, red, silvery, scaled patches on the skin. Also known as inflammatory skin condition, it is seen in both men and women and usually appears in the age of 15-30 years. Heredity factor, abnormality in the metabolism of amino acids and proteins, seasonal changes, injury to the skin and skin infections are some of the causes of psoriasis. The ailment can be cured at home also, using the natural ways.

Home Remedy for Psoriasis

- Simmer 25 grams each of dried burdock seed and chamomile flowers in 600 ml of water, for about 15 minutes. Strain the mixture through a clean cloth, sweeten it with honey and store it in a refrigerator. Have 3 tablespoons of the decoction, 3 to 4 times a day, on a regular basis.

- In a small cup of olive oil, put 2 drops of calendula oil and 1 drop of oregano oil. Rub it on the affected area.
- In 4 cups of water, boil 4 marigold heads, for about 2 minutes. Once cooled, massage the lotion into your scalp. Then, wash the hair with a mild shampoo. Add lemon juice or cider vinegar to the rinsing water to ensure a thorough rinse.
- Mix a cup of freshly prepared bitter gourd juice with a tsp of limejuice. Drink this mixture every day, on an empty stomach, for 4 to 5 days.
- Mud packs are effective in treating psoriasis. Take powdered Fuller's earth and add enough water to form a paste. Apply this paste on the affected area, let it dry and rinse off. It will help remove toxins from your skin.
- Mix Aloe Vera gel and garlic oil in equal proportions. Apply on the affected area. This is a good natural remedy for psoriasis.
- Seawater is beneficial in curing psoriasis. Regular seawater baths as well as application of seawater over the affected parts is one of the best ways of treating psoriasis.
- Wash the affected area to ensure that it is clean. Next, apply cashew nut oil on it and keep it overnight. Wash off in the morning.
- Cabbage leaves act favorably in treating psoriasis. Remove the thick veins of the leaves and wash them thoroughly. Apply on the affected area.
- Hot Epsom salt bath is used to treat psoriasis. Apply olive oil after the Epsom salt bath. It will prove beneficial in curing psoriasis.

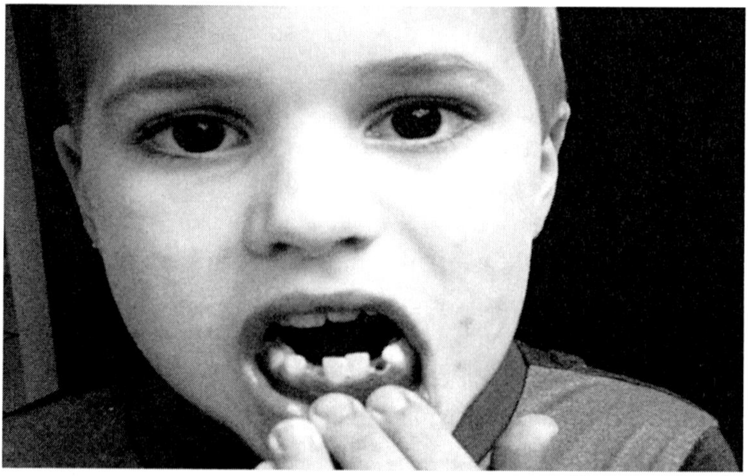

83. Pyorrhea

Periodontitis, more popularly known as pyorrhea, is a condition in which blood and pus comes out from the gums. It affects people of all ages and is basically caused by bacterial activity on the gums that cover the teeth. Constant redness of the gums that aggravates while brushing, flossing or biting into hard foods, presence of blood in the interspaces between the teeth, bad breath, swelling of the gums, recession of the gums, loosening of the teeth from the gums and pain in biting and chewing food are some of the symptoms of pyorrhea. It is the foremost reason for the loss of teeth in old age. Poor nutrition, improper cleaning, drugs, certain medication and infections of the teeth are some of the causes of pyorrhea. However, pyorrhea can be easily treated with natural ways.

Home Remedy for Pyorrhea

- After brushing, take some mustard oil and add a pinch of salt to it. Rub this mixture on the gums, with the tip of your forefinger. An alternative would be to soak cotton ball in mustard oil and rub it on the gums.
- In a bowl of water, immerse some parwal leaves, ginger, black pepper, peepal root and rock salt. Boil the water

until the decoction is ready. Now, strain it with a cloth and allow it to cool. Use this decoction for gargling.

- Boil 4 to 5 bark pieces in a vessel of water, for about half an hour. After the decoction cools down a bit, strain it and use it for gargling. This would be effective in treating pyorrhea.
- Blend 200 ml castor oil and 5 grams camphor in 100 ml honey. Dip one of the ends of a neem twig in it and rub it lightly on your teeth.
- Raw lemon juice is effective in treating pyorrhea. All you need to do is rub the juice over the gums. It would give a tingling sensation, but stop the bleeding.
- Another beneficial remedy will be to gargle with a mouthful of sesame oil. Do this for 10 minutes.
- Take some pieces of the trunk of babul tree and burn them. When they get completely burned, blow off the flame and store it in a cool, dry place. Every morning, take a piece of the burned trunk and dab it with salt. Now, rub the dabbed portion on the teeth. Another alternative would be to dip it in mustard oil before dabbing with salt and applying.
- In a spoonful of pure ghee, mix some camphor and form a paste. Apply this paste over the gums, two times a day.
- Crush some pepper to form a fine powder. Add some salt to it. Now, massage the mixture onto the gums, several times a day. This is an effective way to cure pyorrhea.
- Another effective remedy would be to have guava. Cut a guava into 4 pieces and sprinkle some salt over them. Now, bite each of the pieces and eat them. It might sound foolish but this would smear vitamin C on the teeth, thereby treating pyorrhea.
- Prepare spinach juice and carrot juice and mix the two in equal proportions. Drink this mixture once in a day.

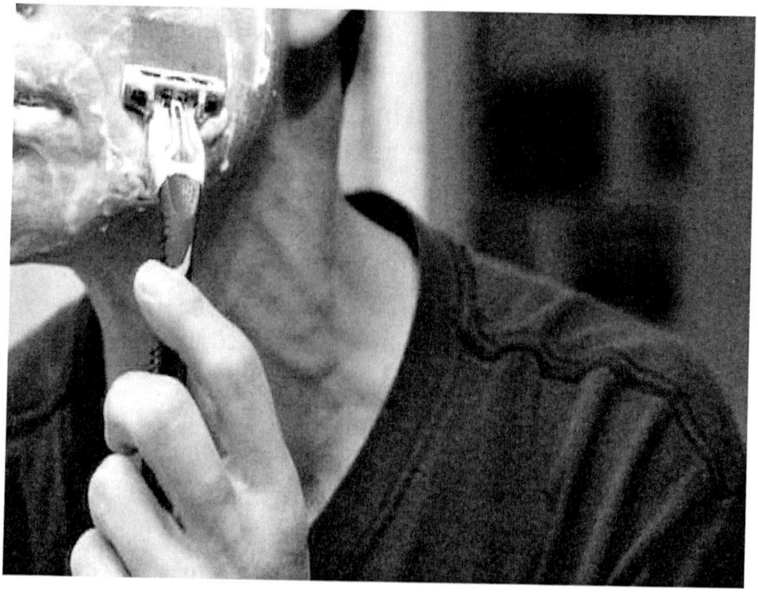

84. Razor Burns

Shaving is a common process that both men and women undertake, to look clean and hygienic. While it makes a person appear neat and tidy, the bad part of it is that it might result in bad patches on the skin, in the form of burns. The small bumps are a result of irritation in the skin, caused by the metal razor. These bumps are known as razor burns. Razor burns usually start from a reddish mild rash, which can lead to itchiness, pain and a burning sensation as well. These burns cause an uncomfortable feeling. However, with little care and the right kind of substances used, they can be avoided as well as healed.

Home Remedy for Razor Burns

- An easy way to treat razor burn at home would be to pat the area with apple cider vinegar.
- In a tsp of sour cream, mix the pulp of 2 strawberries and form a paste. Apply this paste on the affected area, as a

mask, for about 10 minutes. Then, wash the area using lukewarm water. Repeat this twice a week.

- Aloe vera oil is helpful in curing razor burns. Dab the shaved area with cotton ball that has been soaked in the oil.
- Potato is effective in curing razor burns. Peel the skin of a potato and cut it in thin slices. Apply this over the affected area.
- Applying petroleum jelly over the affected area three times a day is an effective way to treat razor burns.
- Before shaving, moisten the area with a wash cloth, dipped in hot water (mixed with lavender essential oil). Pat the skin several times with this. Now, apply a thin layer of moisturizing oil, like avocado or jojoba. This will help you avoid razor burns and also make shaving an easy process.
- Mix 1 tbsp each of dried comfrey leaves and dried calendula flowers in 1/2 cup of witch hazel extract and keep it for 2 weeks. Store this lotion and use it whenever razor burns occur. It usually lasts for about 6 months.
- In ¼ cup of rose water, mix ¼ cup of strained witch hazel. In this, add 1/4 tsp vegetable glycerin, along with 5 drops each of lavender essential oil and sandalwood essential oil. Use it on the affected area. Store it in a cool place and shake it each time before use.
- Shaving in the direction of hair growth is time consuming, but is definitely one of the safest ways to avoid razor burns.

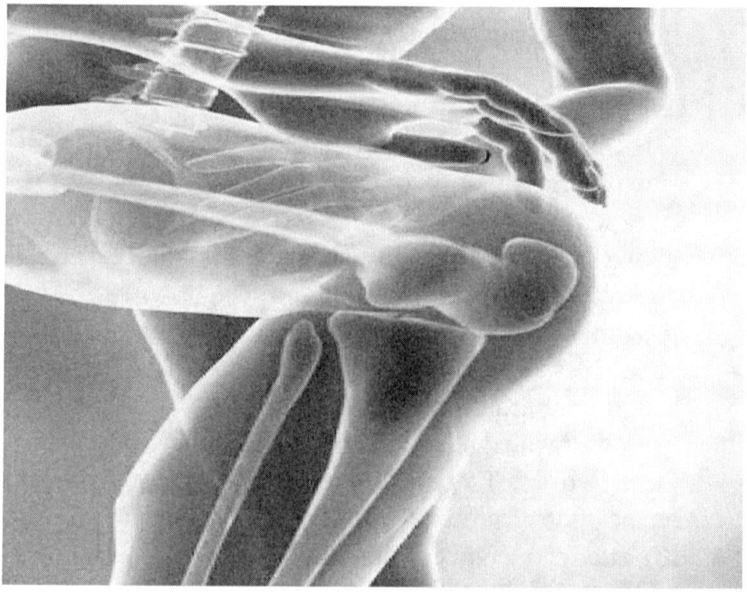

85. Rheumatism

Derived from a Greek word 'rhuema', which means swelling, rheumatism is essentially a condition in which a person experiences severe pain in bone, muscles and joints, along with swelling. It mostly affects people above 45 years of age and is found in both men and women. There are basically two types of rheumatism - muscular rheumatism, which affects the muscles, and articular rheumatism, which affects the joints. Some of the causes of rheumatism are poisoning of blood with acid wastes, physically stressful work, damp weather conditions and acid-alkaline imbalance. Heredity factors, hormonal disorder and infection in teeth are some of the other causes of rheumatism. However, rheumatism can be cured with some natural remedies.

Home Remedy for Rheumatism

- An effective way to treat rheumatism would be to have one or two tsp of raw potato juice before meals.
- Mix 1 tablespoon of cod liver oil in a glass of orange juice. Whip and drink this juice before going to bed.

- In a glass of warm water, dissolve 2 tsp each of apple cider vinegar and honey. Have this concoction once or twice a day.
- Mix carrot juice and lemon juice in equal proportions. Have a large spoonful of this concoction, everyday, to cure rheumatism.
- In two tbsp of water, add one tbsp fresh limejuice. Have this twice a day -in the morning and at night.
- In a pint of warm water, mix juice of three lemons and three tablespoons Epsom salts. Take one tsp of the mixture in the morning and one in the evening.
- Mix oil of wintergreen, chloroform and rubbing alcohol in the ratio of 1:3:12. Once the mixture is prepared, rub it on the affected area.
- In a quarter of cranberry juice, dissolve 4 tsp blackstrap molasses. Drink one glass of this juice everyday, for curing rheumatism.
- Peel some potatoes. Wash 30 grams of this peeling in half a liter of water. Strain the decoction and have it three or four times daily. This is an effective way to treat rheumatism.
- The green stalk of rhubarb is effective in curing rheumatism. Crush this with equal amounts of sugar. Have a tsp of this mixture three or four times everyday.
- Include foods rich in calcium, magnesium and vitamin C in the diet. This would help in treating rheumatism.
- Extract a cup of bitter gourd juice. Mix it with a tsp of honey. Daily dose of this, for three months, would be helpful in treating rheumatism.
- Celery is beneficial in curing rheumatism. You can either use it as a condiment or a fluid extract. 5 to 10 drops of this fluid should be mixed with a glass of hot water. Have this decoction before meals.

- Consuming half a dozen walnuts everyday is beneficial in treating rheumatism. However, make sure you chew them properly.
- In a bucket of warm water, add some rosemary oil. Dip the affected area in this water. This would provide relief from the pain and treat the inflammation as well.

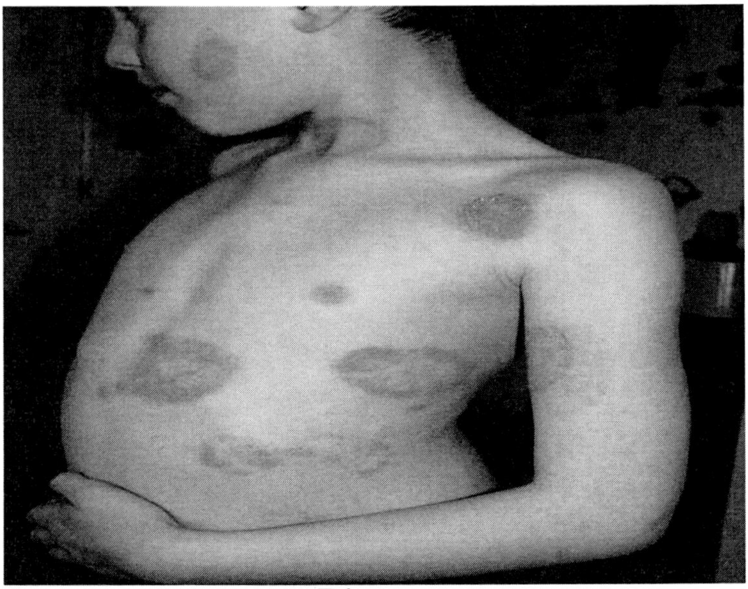

86. Ringworm

Ringworms may infect the human body either in the form of a skin disease or as a parasite that thrives on human body and lies in the intestine. As a fungal infection, it can be found under the fingernails or any place in the body, feet and scalp. It forms a red round spot on the skin and is contagious in nature. Ringworms can be passed from one person to the other by direct skin-to-skin contact or on contact with contaminated articles such as combs, unwashed clothing and shower or pool surfaces. Ringworm patches last on the skin for a maximum of 2 weeks, while the ones on the scalp can extend anywhere between four days to a week. The ringworms that are found in the intestine are generally caused due to weak immune system. Whatever be the type of ringworm infection, it can be treated by resorting to certain natural ways.

Home Remedy for Ringworm

For Ringworm Patches

- Papaya is beneficial in treating ringworm patches. Rub a slice of papaya on the ringworm patches. Another alternative would be to make a paste with the powder of dry papaya seeds and water. Apply this paste over the ringworm patches. Let it dry and then wash off.

- Prepare a paste of mustard seeds and water. Wash the skin using hot water thoroughly before applying this paste over the ringworm patches. Let the paste dry and then rinse it off with cool water.
- Make a paste using the seeds of the herb butea, combined with some lime juice. Apply this past over the affected area and rinse it off after it dries. This is effective way to treat ringworm.
- Extract the juice of the leaves of cassia tree and apply on the affected area. It will help stop the irritation of the skin and lessen the swelling and pain as well. Another way would be make a paste out of the leaves, with water, and apply it on the patches.
- Extract the juice of holy basil and apply it over the affected area. This will prove beneficial in treating ringworm patches.
- The juice of raw turmeric is beneficial, when applied on the patches. You can also consume a mixture of 1 tsp turmeric juice and 1 tsp honey.
- Raw vegetable juice is beneficial in treating ringworm patches. Combine 300 ml carrot juice and 200 ml spinach juice and drink on a daily basis.

For Intestinal Ringworms

- For treating intestinal ringworms, the best bet would be to have ½ cup juice of mint leaves daily. This will be helpful in curing ringworms.
- Drinking 1 oz fresh amla juice everyday, for five days, will prove helpful in destroying worms.

- For children, soak cotton ball in asafetida solution and place it on the anus. This would be helpful in treating ringworms.
- Having tomatoes, sprinkled with black pepper and salt, early in the morning, on an empty stomach, is effective in curing ringworms.
- Two grams of powdered mango kernel, taken with hot water, will be effective in treating ringworms.
- Consuming mulberry fruit is helpful in curing ringworm. The syrup of the fruit is also helpful in killing the worms.

87. Scurvy

Prolonged deficiency of ascorbic acid, also known as vitamin C, in the human body causes scurvy. It is also known as Moeller's disease, Cheadle's disease and Barlow's disease. Scurvy is characterized by darkened gums and loose teeth and is generally seen in people whose diet is low in fresh fruits and green leafy vegetables. The symptoms of scurvy are bleeding gums, joints pain, poor healing capacity of the wounds, liver spots and general weakness of the body. People who spend a lot of time away from the main land (being on sea), children with diet lacking in vitamin C and infants weaned early from their mother's milk are those whom scurvy is likely to strike more. However, the ailment can be treated at home easily, using the natural remedies.

Home Remedy for Scurvy

- Extract the juice of a lemon and mix it with one tsp honey. Now, put this mixture in a glass of warm water. Have this decoction two times a day.
- Indian gooseberry is beneficial in treating scurvy. The fruit of this plant should be eaten regularly. Have four fruits per day, at different periods.
- Another way to treat scurvy would be to mix powdered Indian gooseberry and sugar in equal amounts. Have 1 tsp of this powder, with a glass of milk, every night, before sleeping.

- Include foods rich in Vitamin C, such as oranges, sweet lemons, watermelons, grapefruits, cantaloupes, green leafy vegetables and tomatoes, in your diet.
- In 500 ml of water, boil some leaves of jaundice berry. Keep on boiling until the decoction gets reduced to one-third. Consume this in a dose of 2 to 4 ml, everyday.
- Powdered raw mango, also known as aamchur, is beneficial in treating scurvy. In a glass of water, add ½ tsp of this powder.
- For infants, the best deal would be to give them cow's milk, along with breast milk.
- Potatoes are also beneficial in treating scurvy. Every 100 grams of potato contains approximately 17 mg of Vitamin C. Consuming potatoes will help you cure the ailment.
- Fresh air and sunshine have proven to be beneficial in curing Vitamin C deficiency. Go out and enjoy mingling with nature.

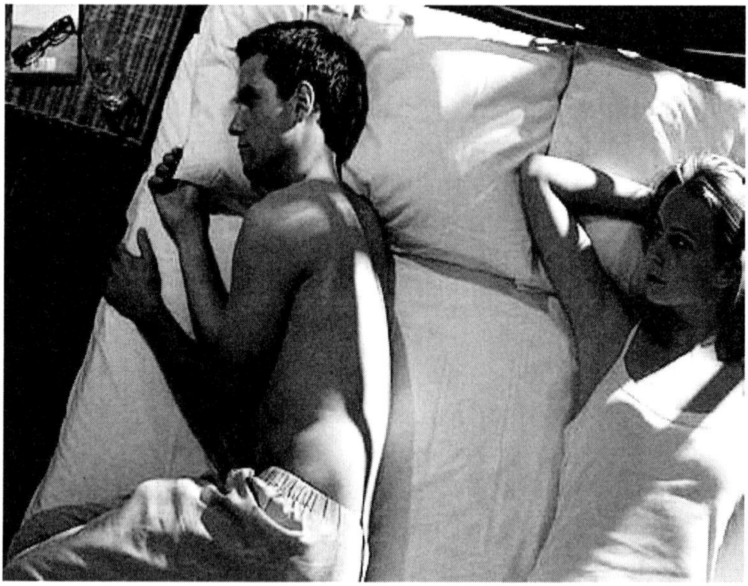

88. Sexual Impotence

Sexual activity is a basic instinct in humans and forms one of the most important aspects of their life. However, there are many people who suffer from sexual dysfunctions. The most commonly found sexual dysfunction in men is impotency. It is a condition in which a person suffers from low sex drive and low erectile functions. One of the main causes of sexual impotence is depression. Devitalized condition of the body system is another reason of sexual impotence. There are three different forms of sexual impotence - primary sexual impotence, secondary sexual impotence and the one concerned with old age. While the third one cannot be treated much, the first two can be cured by resorting to some natural ways.

Home Remedy for Sexual Impotence

- Consuming garlic is one of the best ways to treat sexual impotence. Chew two to three cloves of raw garlic, on a daily basis. In fact, you should include garlic in your regular diet.

- Onion is another very good vegetable to treat sexual impotence. It increases libido and strengthens reproducing organs. White onions are best for this purpose.
- Finely chop about 150 grams of carrots. Consume this, along with a half-boiled egg, dipped in a tablespoon of honey, once everyday. This will help increase sexual stamina.
- Take about 5-10 gm root powder of Ladyfinger in a glass of milk. Add 2 tsp of mishri in this milk and drink it. This will prove helpful in improving sexual vigor.
- Put 15 gm dried roots of asparagus in a glass of milk. Have this milk two times in a day. It will be useful in treating both sexual impotency and premature ejaculation.
- In 250ml of boiled milk, add 15 grams drumstick flowers. Prepare a soup from this decoction. Another effective way to use drumsticks would be to boil 120 gm of the powder of the dry bark in half a liter of water, for about half an hour. Yet another effective way would be to have 30 grams of this powder with a tablespoon of honey. Have this paste 3 times in a day.
- Ginger juice is beneficial in treating sexual impotence. Mix ½ tsp ginger juice with half boiled egg and honey. Have this mixture once every night. It is beneficial in curing impotency, premature ejaculation and spermatorrhoea.
- Dry fruits are effective in curing sexual impotency. Pound and mix equal quantities of dates, almonds, pistachios and quince seeds. 100 grams of this mixture, consumed on a daily basis, is said to increase sexual power.
- Wash 30 grams of black raisins in lukewarm water. Eat them with a glass of warm milk, daily. Increase the quantity by 50 grams after some time.

- Mix jambul fruit (Indian herb) with milk and add a little honey to it. Consume this mixture to treat impotence.
- Some of the items that help normalize hormonal imbalance and boost sexual craving are chickweed, ginseng, plantain and safflower. Include them in your diet.
- For female sterility, dry the roots of banyan tree and powder them into fine particles. Take about 20 gm of this powder with milk, in a ratio of 1:5. Have this for 3 consecutive nights after the menstrual cycle.
- Powder winter cherry herb. Consume 6 grams of this powder, with a cup of milk, for 5 to 6 days after menstruation.
- Including lots of seeds, fruits, nuts, grains, fresh green vegetables and fresh fruits in the diet is helpful in treating sexual impotence.

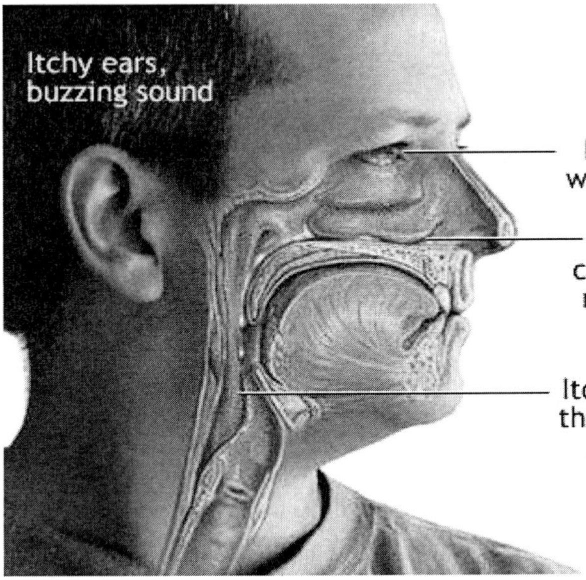

89. Sinusitis

Sinusitis can be described as an inflammation of the mucous membrane lining the para-nasal sinuses. In simple terms, it can be defined as the over secretion of mucus by the membranes lining the nose and throat. The most common symptoms of sinusitis are constant or excessive sneezing, low grade fever, running nose, headaches, blockage of one or both nostrils, and pressure around the eyes, head, and face. Lack of appetite and difficulty in breathing are the other symptoms of sinusitis. However, sinusitis can be cured by resorting to some natural ways of treatment.

Home Remedy for Sinusitis

- Raw vegetable juice is beneficial in treating sinusitis. Combine 300 ml of carrot juice, 100 ml of cucumber juice, 100 ml of beet juice and 200 ml of spinach juice and drink on a daily basis.
- Consuming fruits rich in Vitamin A is effective in sinusitis. One of the richest sources of the vitamin is mango. So,

patients suffering from sinus should have lots of mangoes. Other food products rich in Vitamin A include pumpkin, leafy vegetables, egg yolk, tomatoes, papaya, carrots, curd and whole milk.

- Roast 100 grams of cumin seeds and mix them with 200 grams of pure ghee. Consume daily. It is one of the most effective ways to cure sinusitis.
- Take a tsp of black cumin seeds and tie them in a thin cloth. Inhaling from the cloth would be effective in reducing sinusitis.
- Boil a tsp of fenugreek seeds in half a glass of water, until the decoction reduces to half. Consuming 3 to 4 cups of this tea would help in expelling all the toxins, increasing the perspiration rate and thereby reducing fever, along with sinusitis.
- Pungent smelling vegetables, like onion and garlic, are helpful in curing sinusitis. Inhaling their smell would also prove to be beneficial.
- Steam is effective in curing sinusitis. It opens the nasal passage by draining the sinuses and making mucous flow easy.
- Avoid cold items and oily stuff. They trigger the upper respiratory diseases, instead of lessening them.
- Gargling with salted lukewarm water is beneficial in treating sinusitis. For this, add a pinch of salt in a glass of lukewarm water and gargle with it.
- Prepare ginger or cinnamon tea and drink it when it is slightly on the hotter side. It is helpful in curing sinusitis.

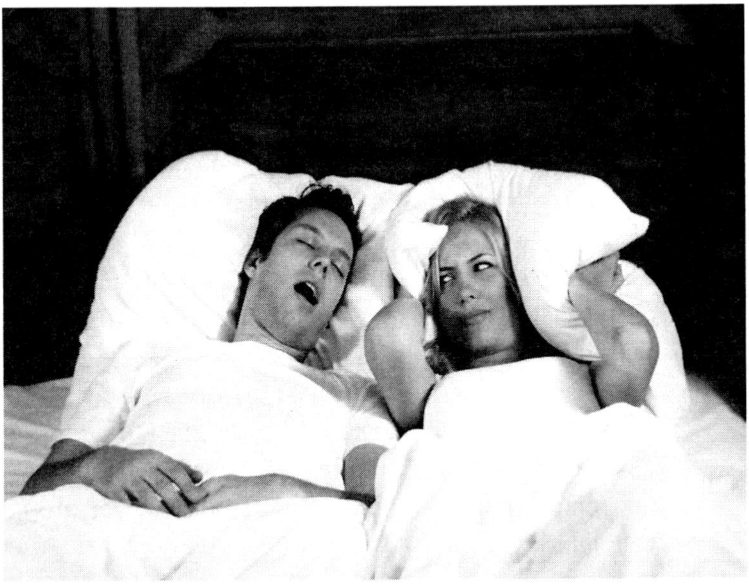

90. Snoring

Snoring is the sound produced, while sleeping, due to the vibration in the respiratory structures. In this situation, the air movement gets obstructed while breathing, resulting in the sound. The throat or pharynx is a muscular tube that relaxes and decreases in size when a person is sleeping. For some people, this narrowing is enough to cause vibration of soft tissues in the pharynx. Some of the causes of snoring include muscle tone of the tongue, blockage of airway, age factor, alcoholic beverages, certain medications and sheer physical exhaustion. While the sound produced while sleeping is the only symptom of snoring, it is, at times, accompanied by heavy breathing as well. Snoring can, however, be treated at home also.

Home Remedy for Snoring

- One of the best ways to stop snoring would be to lose weight. This might surprise you, but weight loss reduces and even ends snoring.

- Another way to stop snoring would be to lessen, better stop, smoking. It is said that smoking causes increased nasal congestion and mucous in the throat area.
- Alcohol causes relaxation in the soft tissues and muscles in the throat, leading to snoring. Reducing the intake of alcohol can lessen, or even stop, snoring.
- The ideal posture while sleeping would be on the sides. This would reduce the intensity of sound created while snoring.
- Olive oil is said to reduce snoring. Take 2 to 3 sips of it before going to bed. This would lessen the noise and also stop snoring after some time.
- Follow a regular sleep routine. Sleep at fixed times and get up at the same time. This is believed to reduce snoring.
- In boiling water, place a bunch of sage and let it steep. Allow it to cool. Before going to bed, strain this mixture and gargle with the liquid. This will prove effective in reducing snoring.
- Avoid having heavy meals or foods that are too spicy or oily, in dinner. They tend to aggravate the problem of snoring.

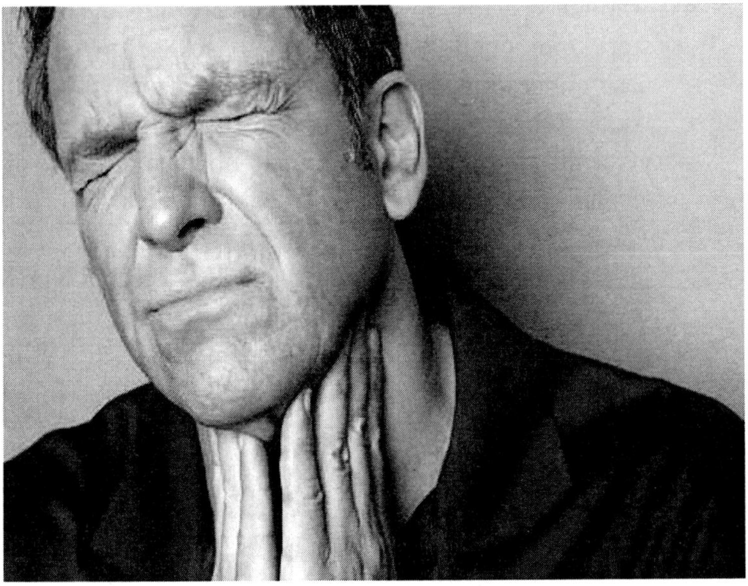

91. Sore Throat

Sore throat is an inflammation or swelling in the pharynx i.e. at the back of the throat. Often caused by a viral infection, sore throat is the result of cold, cough or flu. Other causes of sore throat include tonsillitis, mumps, sinusitis, measles, diphtheria, leukemia, excessive smoking, talking loudly and shouting. Some of the most common symptoms of sore throat are irritation of throat, chills and fever, pain, swollen and tender lymph glands and difficulty in swallowing. Though sore throat is generally harmless, it can cause serious problems if prolonged. Still, sore throats can be effectively treated at home, using the natural therapies.

Home Remedy for Sore Throat

- The most effective way to cure sore throat would be to mix 4 cloves of garlic, 1 tbsp of honey and 1/8 tsp of cayenne. Have 1 tsp of this mixture, everyday, during sore throat. Make sure to chew it well, before swallowing.

- In a cup of water, put some Holy Basil leaves. Boil this concoction, allow it to cool and strain well. You can either drink it or use it for gargling.
- A simple remedy for treating sore throat would be to gargle with lukewarm water. Add some salt to it, before gargling. This would surely provide relief.
- In a pint of boiling water, add 1 or 2 tsp dried chamomile blossoms. Let them steep well and then strain the water. Have a cup of this decoction, every few hours, during sore throat.
- Another effective home remedy for sore throat would be to mix a tsp each of apple cider vinegar and honey, along with a pinch of cayenne pepper and extracted juice of 1/4th lemon, in a cup of hot water. Stir well before drinking. Have this mixture 4 times in a day.
- Boil a glass of water. In it, add a pinch of powdered cloves, a pinch of pepper powder and 1 tsp honey. Drink this concoction once in a day, preferably early morning. This is an effective way to cure sore throat.
- Fenugreek seeds are beneficial in treating sore throat. In a glass of lukewarm water, add some fenugreek seeds and let them steep for sometime. Strain the water and gargle with it, to cure sore throat.
- In a pint of boiling water, add 2 sprigs of coarsely chopped parsley, 3 whole spice cloves, 1 tsp of powdered myrrh and 1/4 tsp of powdered goldenseal. Let the water simmer for sometime, cool it and then strain the decoction. Use it for gargling.
- Take a cup with a lid and put some honey in it. Now, cut an onion slice and soak it in the honey. Put on the lid and keep aside for an hour. Have a tsp of this honey every few hours.

- Another beneficial method to get relief from sore throat would be to drink a glass of warm water, with lemon juice and some honey added to it.
- Take a lemon and cut it into two halves. In one of the pieces, sprinkle some salt and black pepper. Press it with a knife so that the pepper and salt penetrates in. Now, warm this lime piece and lick it. Have this twice or thrice a day, to get immediate relief from sore throat.
- Barberry Tincture is effective in curing sore throat. Take 1/4th cup water and add 15 to 20 drops of the tincture to it. Have this water thrice daily, for 10 days.
- In 600 ml of water, add 25 grams fresh sage water and 1/4th tsp cayenne. Give it a boil and allow it to cool. Now, strain this decoction and drink once in a day.
- Make tea by putting a tsp of dried red sage in one cup of boiling water. Cover it with a lid and leave for 10 minutes. Now, strain this mixture and add a few drops of vinegar to it. You can either drink it as tea or use it for gargling.

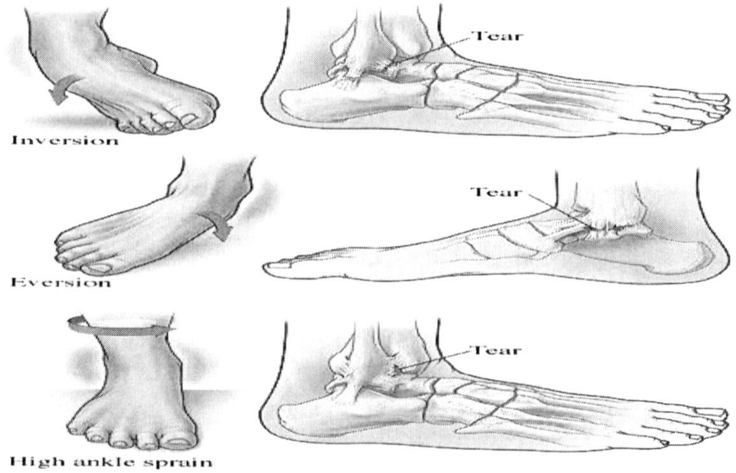

92. Sprain

Wear and tear of the ligaments is a common phenomenon, especially when a person indulges in regular physical activity. A sprain can be described as an injury in which the tissues around the injured joint get torn. These tissues, better known as ligaments, are extremely soft in nature. They connect two or more bones together to form a joint. During a sprain, one or more ligaments get worn out and tear apart. Wrists, ankles and knees are the areas most susceptible to sprains. Some of the common causes of sprain are sudden fall, a forceful blow to the body, twisting, stepping on an uneven surface, lifting heavy objects and over-stretching of the ligaments. Though it is not a fracture, sprain can be just as painful.

Home Remedy for Sprain

- The most effective way to treat sprain would be to apply cold compress on the area and cover it with a bandage.
- For a foot sprain, the best bet would be to put a tbsp of black coffee in the bandage and wrap the hurt foot with it.
- A simple way to get relief from pain and cure sprain would be to soak the outer leaves of a cabbage in water. Now,

wrap the sprained area with these leaves and let them remain there for about 10 to 15 minutes.

- In a bowl of warm water, put a few drops of lavender oil. Soak the sprained area in this water.
- A popular home remedy for sprain is to massage the area with a mixture of almond oil and garlic oil.
- Chop onions and wrap them in a muslin cloth. Place the cloth on the affected area for sometime.
- In a cup of sunflower oil, mix 1 tsp of camphor oil. Massage the affected area with this oil mixture. It would provide immense relief from the pain.
- Another effective oil combination would comprise of a mixture of 2 tbsp sunflower oil and 1 tbsp turpentine oil. Store this mixture in a glass jar and massage the sprained area with it, on a daily basis.
- An effective way to cure the pain experienced during sprain would be to have lots of pineapple but you must ensure that you have fresh pineapples since canned and processed foods may lose a lot of their nutritional values.
- A simple way to cure sprain would be to give the affected area a hot Epsom salt bath.
- In case of immense pain, take a glass of warm milk and add some turmeric powder to it. Have this milk two times a day. It would provide instant relief.
- In a tsp of honey, add 1 tsp of lime juice. Massage this mixture on the affected area to treat sprains.
- Prepare a paste by blending together lime leaves and butter. Apply this paste over the sprained area and leave it there for sometime. This would help heal the sprain.
- To get relief from the pain experienced during sprain, add five drops of thyme oil to your bathing water and have a hot tub bath.

93. Stomach Ache

One of the most common ailments, stomach ache can be experienced anywhere in the area that falls between the chest and groin. This pain can vary from being mild to moderate and severe. Men, women and children, all are susceptible to stomach pain. Some of the major causes of the ache are chronic constipation, indigestion, excessive gas, food poisoning, ulcers, appendicitis, inflammation of the gallbladder, kidney stones, urinary tract infections and hernia.

Home Remedy for Stomach Ache

- One of the most effective home remedies for stomach ache would be to mix 1 tsp each of mint juice and limejuice. To it, add a few drops of ginger juice and a pinch of black salt. Drink this mixture to alleviate pain.
- Grate a small piece of ginger and extract its juice. Apply this juice on the bottom of the belly and massage it gently. This will be effective in curing stomach ache.
- If the stomach ache is due to acidity, the best bet would be to drink plain soda water. It would provide instant relief from the pain.
- In 50 ml water, mix 2 tsp lemon juice and 1 gram rock salt powder. Have this mixture three times a day.
- Take dry ginger, black pepper, roasted cumin seeds, dry mint leaves, coriander, asafetida, garlic and rock salt in equal quantities. Grind them well and make a fine powder. Have 1 tsp of this mixture, along with a glass of warm water, after meals.

- Taking three grams each of carom seeds and rock salt or common salt, along with a glass of warm water, helps in relieving a person from stomach ache.
- In half a cup of warm water, add a tsp each of ginger juice and castor oil. Have this mixture two times a day, to get relief from stomach ache.
- In a cup of water, add 20 grams aniseeds. Keep it overnight and strain the mixture the next morning. Drink it to get relief from pain.
- Mix one gram of rock salt and two grams of dried and crushed celery leaves. Eat it to get instant relief from stomach ache.
- Grind three grams of tender tamarind leaves, with enough water, to make a paste. Once it turns into a liquefied form, add a gram of rock salt. Drink this mixture to get relief from stomach ache.
- Combine 2 tsp lemon juice and 1 tsp ginger juice. Add ¼ tsp sugar to this mixture and have it two times in a day.
- Pomegranates are helpful in treating stomach ache. In a bowl of pomegranate seeds, sprinkle some salt and black pepper. Eat the seeds, while making sure to chew them properly.
- Grind bael (Aegle marmelos) and form a pulp. Mix it in a glass of freshly prepared buttermilk. Stir it well before drinking.
- Prepare a paste of fenugreek seeds. Now, add this paste to a bowl of curd. This is one of the most effective ways to treat stomach cramps and pain.
- In half a liter of water, add 2 grams each of black currants and fennel seeds and keep it overnight. The next morning, mash the contents in water and add a gram of sugar. Have this concoction daily, in the morning, to get relief from chronic stomach ache.

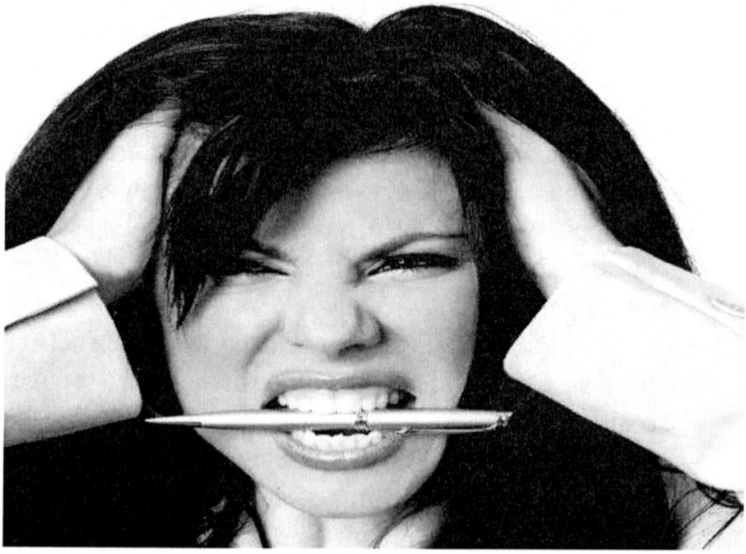

94. Stress

Stress is the term given to the difficulty that the body faces while combating a physical or emotional threat, be it actual or imagined. Some of the common symptoms of stress include irritability, muscular tension, inability to concentrate and a variety of physical reactions, such as headaches and accelerated heart rate. Stress is not always harmful. Sometimes, it helps a person perform better and achieve his/her goals. However, excess of stress can work negatively, hampering the work and lifestyle of a person.

Home Remedy for Stress

- The most effective way to treat stress would be to chew 10-20 leaves of Holy Basil everyday.
- Another effective home remedy would be to prepare a decoction of Holy Basil leaves. For this, add 20 to 25 leaves in half a liter of water. Boil this decoction until it gets reduced to half. Strain the mixture and drink it while it's still warm.

- Prepare a paste with dry ginger and water/ milk. Apply this on your forehead. Its cooling properties will help ease off the stress a bit.
- Take some betel leaves and wash them in water. Place the leaves on the forehead and leave them there for sometime. This is likely to bring relief from stress.
- Bishop's Weeds (Ajwain) are effective in treating stress. Put a handful of the seeds in a handkerchief and sniff them for sometime.
- Exercise, yoga and meditation are likely to relieve a person from stress, provided you indulge in them on a regular basis.
- Include lots of green leafy vegetables, fruits, salads, whole wheat grains, beans, grams, sprouts, eggs, cheese, soybeans and fresh curd in your diet.
- Cut down on the consumption of junk foods, oily and over fried foods, sugar, sweets and alcohol.
- It is advisable to have 5 almonds, along with a glass of warm milk, every morning, to get relief from stress.
- Sage is valuable in the treatment of stress. In a cup of boiling water, add a tsp of dried sage leaves. Now, cover the cup with a lid and let the leaves steep for sometime. Strain the decoction and add honey to it. Drink this liquid while it's still warm.
- Have foods rich in Vitamin A and Vitamin B. They would provide your body the nutrients required to combat stress.

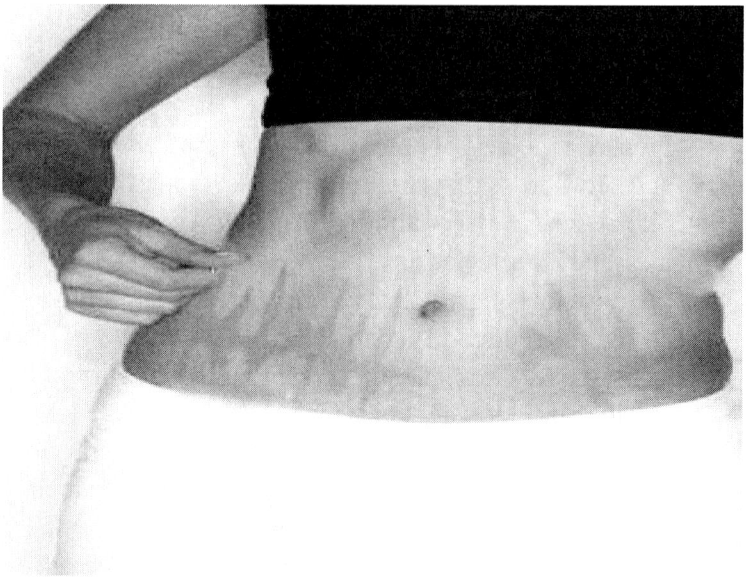

95. Stretch Marks Removal

Stretch marks can be described as lines on the skin surface, with an off-color hue. Such lines are mainly found in the abdominal wall, below the umbilicus, but can also occur over the thighs and breasts. While pregnancy is the predominant cause of stretch marks, other reasons include gain or loss in weight, rapid growth (especially in adolescents), heredity factors, stress and changes in physical conditions. Medically termed as striae gravidarum, stretch marks are initially pink in color, but change to white later on. Mistaken for scars, they are essentially a flattened, thin epidermis, overlying gaps in the dermis, left by stretched or torn elastin fibers. Given below are some of the home remedies for getting rid from them easily.

Home Remedy for Stretch Marks Removal

- One of the simplest, yet effective home remedies for stretch marks would be to apply lavender oil on the marks, three times a day.

- Another home remedy would be to apply Aloe Vera gel on the marks. They would initially, lighten and finally, remove the marks from the body.
- Prepare a mixture by adding seven drops of lavender oil and a few drops of chamomile oil to an ounce of carrier oil (avocado, sweet almond or jojoba oil). Use it to massage the affected area.
- Includes lots of green leafy vegetables, tomatoes, liver and dairy products in your diet.
- Consume seeds and nuts that contain zinc. They will prove effective in removing stretch marks.
- In a blender, mix ½ cup olive oil, ¼ cup Aloe vera gel, liquid from 6 Vitamin E capsules and liquid from 4 Vitamin A capsules. Store it in a container and place it in the refrigerator. Apply this mixture wherever stretch marks appear.
- Aroma oil is beneficial in treating stretch marks problem. Apply some of this oil on the stretch marks and massage well.
- Rub the affected area with apricot scrub. This is likely to remove the stretch marks gradually.
- Cocoa butter is beneficial in treating stretch marks. Apply it two times a day, in the morning as well as in the evening, over the affected area. This would help remove the marks.

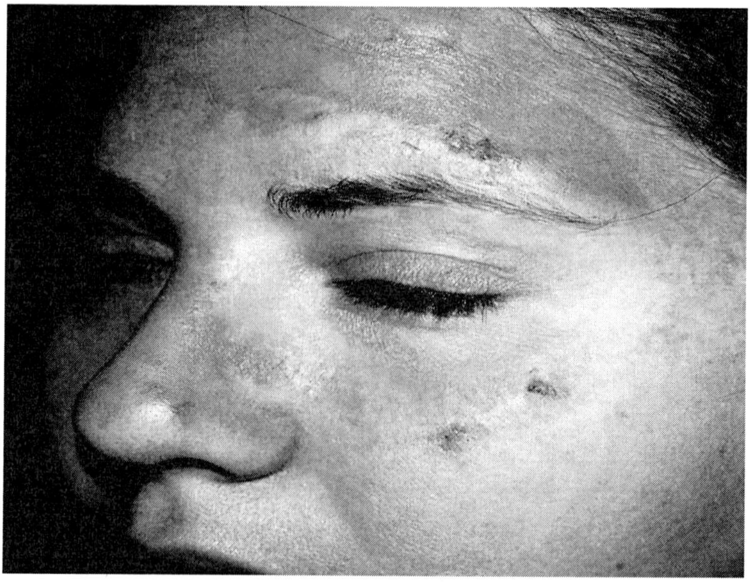

96. Sunburn

Sunburn is the name of a burn that results from exposure to ultraviolet radiation and results in the inflammation of the skin. Over exposure to sun rays and ultraviolet light are the most prevalent causes of sunburn. Though the problem does not seem to be too severe, in worst cases, it might lead to death and even permanent disability. Possibility of getting skin cancer is also not ruled out. Some of the symptoms of sunburn include pain, heat and redness in the affected area, which also becomes tender to touch.

Home Remedy for Sunburn

- An effective remedy for treating sunburn would be to apply a cloth dipped in milk on the affected area. This would provide relief from the burn.
- Another effective remedy would be to rub the affected area with mustard oil. Apart from removing the burn, it would also provide relief from the itching.

- Apply sliced cucumber or potato on the sun-burnt area. They would provide a soothing effect to the area.
- Lavender oil is beneficial in treating sunburn. Apply it on the affected area to get relief from the pain and itching.
- Take some sandalwood powder and water. Prepare a paste from the two and apply on the affected area. This is sure to relieve a person from the burning sensation.
- In a bowl, mix tomato juice and buttermilk, in the ratio of 1:6. Apply this on the sun burnt area. Wash it after 30 minutes.
- Mix equal proportions of olive oil and vinegar and apply on the affected area. Wash this after about an hour. This will bring relief from the sunburn.
- Another effective home remedy would be to mix barley flour, honey and raw egg, to make a paste. Apply this paste over the sun-burnt area and wash off after sometime.
- Take some water in a bowl and put lettuce leaves in it. Place it on flame and bring to a boil. Once it has cooled down, strain the liquid and apply it on the affected area, using cotton balls.
- Before bathing, pour a cup of white cider vinegar into the bathtub and enjoy a long bath. This would provide relief from the sunburn.
- Mix wheat flour, milk and olive oil to make a paste. Apply this paste on the affected area. After the paste dries, wash it off.
- Applying Aloe Vera gel on the affected area proves beneficial in treating sunburns.
- In a blender, mix 2 tomatoes and 1 cucumber and make a puree. To this, add a few drops of lemon juice. Apply this paste over the suntanned and sun-burnt skin. Once dry, dab the puree once again. Repeat the process three times.

It would help remove the burn and also add a glow to the skin.

- Boil some cabbage leaves and mash them. Apply the mashed cabbage over the tanned and sun-burnt areas. Wash off it after 15 minutes.
- Rubbing green gourd on the affected areas, 3 to 4 times a day, is helpful in removing the sunburn.
- A mixture of honey and lime is effective in treating sunburn. In 2 tbsp of honey, add a few drops of lemon juice. Apply this over the affected area. It would help lighten the tan and ease off the pain as well.
- In 3 tablespoons of milk, add 1 tbsp of turmeric powder. Apply this all over the affected area. Once dry, wet it a little and rub in circular motions, before rinsing it off with cool water.

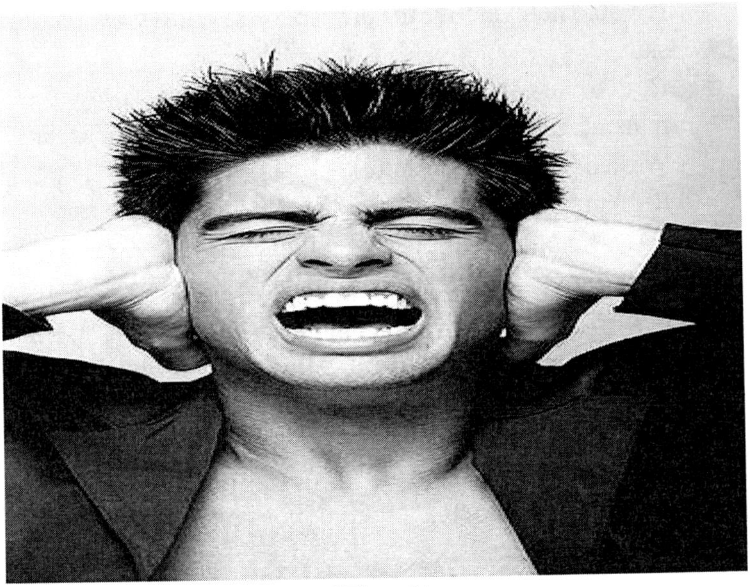

97. Tinnitus

Tinnitus is a buzzing sound that can be heard in one or both of the ears. The sound may either be consistent or come and go at varied intervals. There are basically two types of tinnitus - objective and subjective. In case of objective tinnitus, not only will the affected person hear a buzzing sound, but those around him would also hear the sound coming from his ears. On the other hand, subjective tinnitus patients will experience the buzzing sound all alone. Damage in the ears, age and presence of any waxy particles inside the ear are some of the reasons of tinnitus. The most common symptoms of the ailment include hissing or buzzing sound inside the ears. These sounds coincide with the heartbeats of the patient. As a result of tinnitus, apart from losing on sleep, the affected person also fails to concentrate on work.

Home Remedy for Tinnitus

- An effective home remedy for tinnitus would be to put 20-40 mg of Maidenhair tree extract inside the ears.

- For people who suffer from tinnitus because of loud noise, the best option would be to wear ear plugs.
- When suffering from tinnitus, it is advisable to avoid saturated fats, processed foods, sugar and salts.
- Coffee, tea, sweet foods and refined alcohol, all add to the tinnitus problem. It is advisable to avoid these foods and beverages.
- Include lots of fruits and vegetables, garlic, kelp and sea vegetables in your diet. Have food rich in protein, vitamin A, vitamin B, vitamin E, zinc and choline.
- Mix a tsp each of salt and glycerin in a pint of warm water. Use this liquid as a nasal spray, spraying it in each nostril until the solution drains to the throat.
- Exercising regularly is a good way to tackle tinnitus problem.
- Wearing earplugs is a good way to cure tinnitus at home. The earplugs can be of any variety, such as rubber, foam or moldable wax ones.
- Have lots of fresh pineapple, as it reduces the inflammation in your ear, thereby curing tinnitus.
- Chewing dry fruits helps enhance the blood circulation, thereby acting beneficially in solving tinnitus.
- Taking hot and cold foot baths, alternatively, proves effective in treating tinnitus.

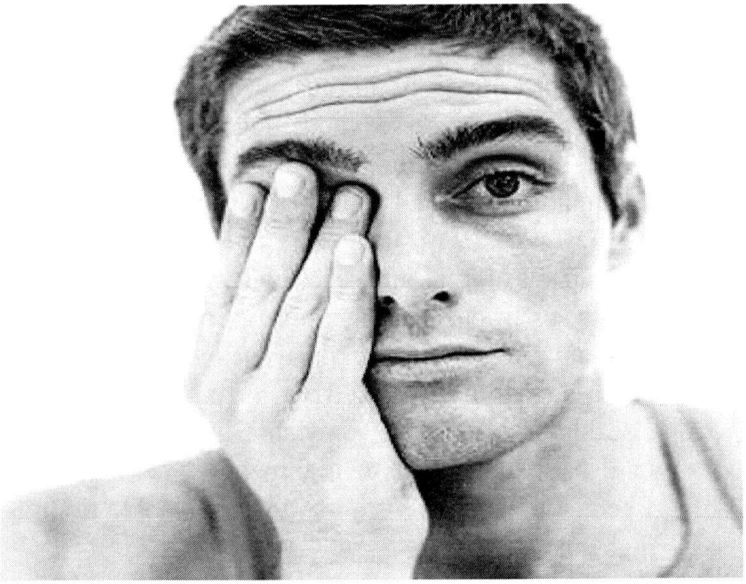

98. Tired Eyes

'Tired eyes' is one of the problems frequently occurring in the present-day world. In this condition, along with puffiness around the eyes, a person also suffers from heaviness in the head. Lack of sleep is one of the primary causes of tired eyes. Other causes include allergy, eyestrain, fatigue, conjunctivitis, excessive crying, inadequate supply of oxygen to the cornea and pollution. Its symptoms are heaviness in eyes, burning sensation, irritation and redness of the eyes. Tired eyes can, however, be treated at home, using the natural ways.

Home Remedy for Tired Eyes

- One of the simplest home remedies for tired eyes would be to place two spoons in the freezer. Take them out when they are cold and place them under the eyes to reduce puffiness. Do not freeze the spoons.

- Another effective method would be to dip cotton balls in tea water. Place the cotton on the eyelids and leave it there for sometime.
- Take a cucumber and cut it into slices. Place the sliced cucumber on your eyelids, to get relief from the puffiness.
- An effective option would be to wash the eyes regularly with cold water. This would help the eyes relax and also remove any kind of tiredness.
- In a small bowl of cold milk, dip a cotton ball and place it over the eyelids. This would remove all the puffiness.
- In a bowl of water, add a few drops of lavender oil. Soak a cotton ball in this and place it over the eyelids.
- Soak a cotton ball in a bowl, containing water, and a few drops of perfume. Keep the soaked cotton on your eyelids, for a few minutes.
- Place a strawberry, kept in the refrigerator for a few minutes, on the eyelids. This will be beneficial in treating tired eyes.
- Boil 2 cups of water. In it, add a small amount of boric acid. Once cooled, use the solution to wash the eyes for quick relief.

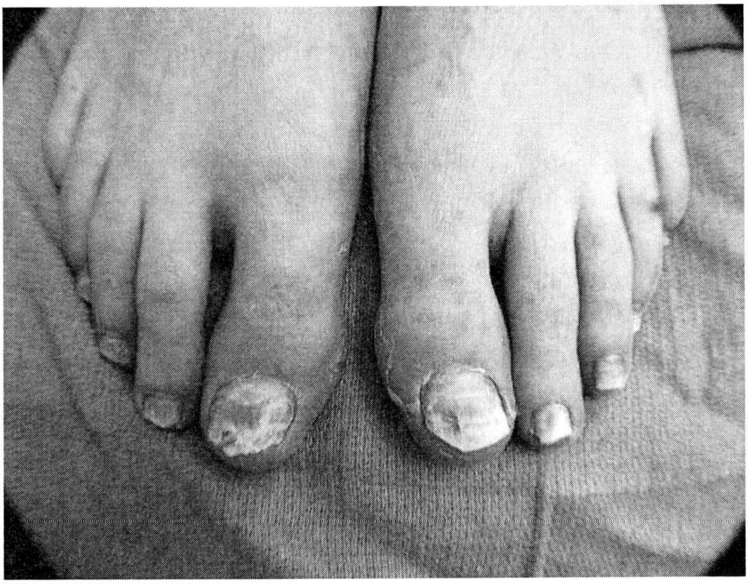

99. Toe Nail Fungus

Toe nail fungus is the result of infection caused by tiny micro-organisms. Also known as Onychomycosis, the fungi grows in the warm and moist fingernails. As the fungi growth increases, it makes the nails hard and brittle and also leads to discoloration. Though toe nail fungus is not painful in the initial stages, it starts hurting later on. Some of the causes of toe nail fungus are a break in the nail, tight-fitting shoes, multiple small cuts in the skin and damp shoes and socks. The fungus causes the toenails to get flaked, brittle and chipped. They also start emitting a bad smell. However, the fungus can be treated at home, using certain home remedies.

Home Remedy for Toe Nail Fungus

- Tea tree oil is effective in treating toe nail fungus. Dip a cotton ball in the oil and rub the toe nail two times a day - once in the morning and the second time while going to bed at night.

- Listerine mouthwash is helpful in treating toe nail fungus. Soak your toes in the mouthwash for about 20 minutes. Its medicinal properties would help control the fungal growth.
- Fill a bucket with equal proportion of water and natural apple cider vinegar. Soak your feet in the bucket for 15 to 20 minutes. Thereafter, dry your toenails thoroughly.
- Mix equal amounts of lavender oil and tea tree oil. Soak a cotton ball in this mixture and dab the toe nail with it, 2 to 3 times in a day. This would be effective in treating toe nail fungus.
- In a tsp of olive oil, add 2 drops of oregano essential oil. Apply this mixture on the affected area. It would help provide relief from toe nail fungus.
- Fill a bucket with equal proportion of water and vinegar. Soak your feet in this combination for 20 minutes. Now, dry the toes with a towel and wipe them with a super absorbent paper. Repeat the process two times a day.
- Another helpful home remedy for toe nail fungus would be to soak the feet in rubbing alcohol, for about 20 minutes.
- Soak your feet in a tub filled with equal proportions of water and Hydrogen Peroxide (3%), for about 15 minutes. After this, dry the feet completely.
- Include lots of probiotics food, such as yogurt and kefir, in your diet. This would help your body get rid of the fungus.
- Make a paste with turmeric powder and water. Apply this paste on your toe nail. Rinse it off when it dries and then properly dry your feet.
- Peel an onion and cut it into slices. Rub the affected toenail with the onion slices for sometime. This is an effective way to treat the fungal infection.

- Another effective home remedy would be to soak a cotton ball in concentrated lime juice. Rub the cotton on the affected toenail.
- It is advisable to wash the feet properly after visiting public places, like swimming pools, spas, showers and locker rooms.
- Avoid sharing towels, washcloths, shoes or any other personal items of people who have already contracted this disease.

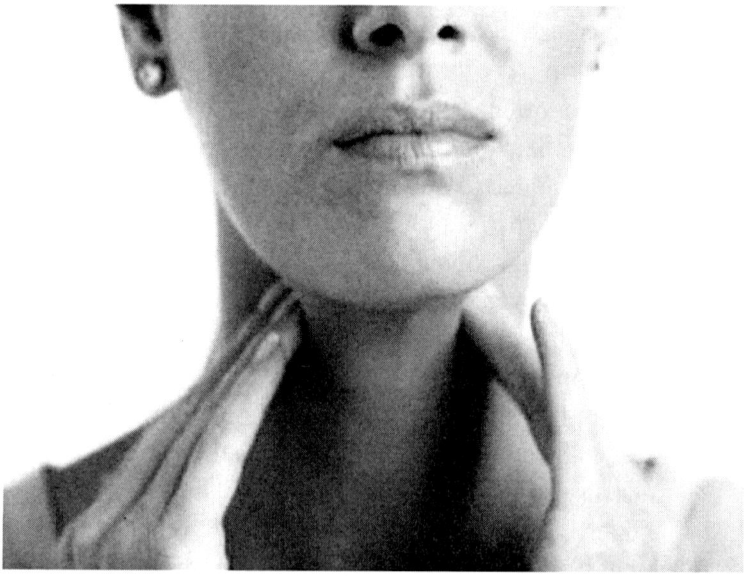

100. Tonsillitis

Tonsils are lymph nodes, located on both sides of the throat. Tonsillitis can be described as a bacterial or viral infection that affects these lymph nodes. This infection results in enlargement of the tonsils. Tonsillitis can be of varying degrees of seriousness - mild, moderate and severe. In case of chronic tonsillitis, enlargement of the tonsils is often accompanied with repeated attacks of infection. A contagious disease by nature, tonsillitis can spread very quickly from one person to another. Some of the most common symptoms of tonsillitis are sore throat, fever, pain in the tonsils (especially when swallowing), runny nose, nasal congestion, coughing and sneezing. The ailment can, however, be treated at home, using natural remedies.

Home Remedy for Tonsillitis

- One of the best home remedies for tonsillitis includes a glass of warm water with four teaspoons of honey, a quarter teaspoon of common salt and a fresh lime squeezed in it. Drink it twice in a day.

- Another effective remedy would be to drink a glass of boiled milk, with a pinch of turmeric powder and pepper powder added to it, before sleeping. Have this for three nights in a row.
- Combination of carrot, beet and cucumber juice is beneficial in curing tonsillitis. Mix 300 ml of carrot juice, 100 ml of beet juice, and 100 ml of cucumber juice and drink once in a day.
- In 50ml of milk, boil 12 gm of Viola odorata flowers. Strain the milk, cool it and drink. The strained residue is also useful in treating tonsillitis. Fry it in a little clarified butter and wear it around the throat, as a poultice, at night.
- In half a liter of water, add 2 tbsp fenugreek seeds and simmer it for half an hour. Let it cool for sometime. Strain the water and gargle with it twice a day. It would be helpful in treating tonsillitis.
- In a grinder, mix equal quantities of mustard, horseradish seeds, jute seeds, flaxseeds, barley and radish seeds. Make a paste out of the mixture and apply it over the tonsils.
- Burn a few twigs of water hyacinth plant, to produce ashes. Put the ashes in mustard oil and apply it over the tonsils. This is a good way to reduce inflammation.
- Soak the roots of white pea in water. Grind them after a few minutes. Drink this water every morning and then eat a chapatti, smeared with ghee.
- Scoop out the pulp of bitter tumbi. Now, fill the kernel of the fruit, from which the pulp has been removed, with water and keep aside for few hours. Drink a little of this water, everyday, for a week. This is an effective way to cure tonsillitis.

- Another useful home remedy would be to boil some dry figs and grind them. Add water to it, to make a paste. Apply it over the throat.
- In a bowl of water, add a portion of babul tree bark and let it boil. Allow it to simmer for 20 minutes. Once cool, strain the decoction and use it for gargling.
- An effective home remedy would be to cut a lemon into two halves. Sprinkle some black pepper and salt on one of the halves and press it inside with a spoon. Keep licking the lemon till the entire juice has been extracted. Repeat the process two times a day.
- Consuming a diet comprising entirely of fruits, for three to four days, would help in treating the tonsillitis.

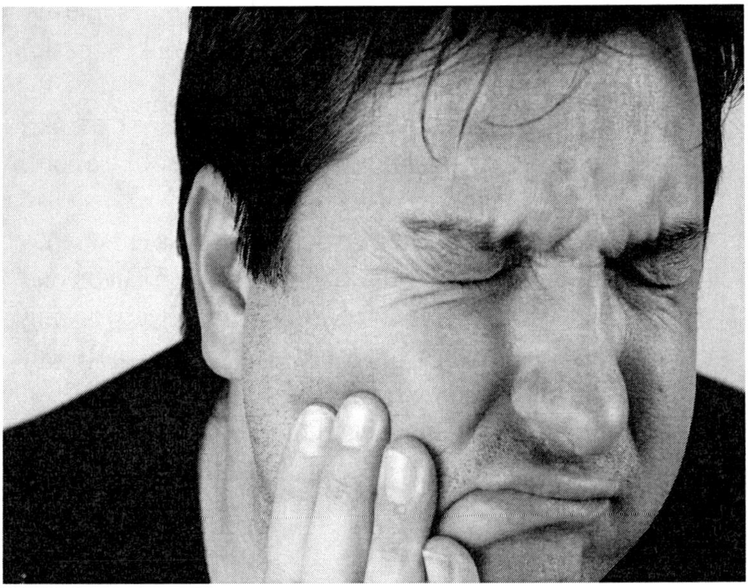

101. Toothache

Toothache can be described as a sensation of pain or soreness either in or around the tooth. It causes inflammation, irritation, swelling and reddening of the area around the affected tooth. The present-day lifestyle, full of stress and unhealthy eating habits, has made toothache a common problem. Some of the reasons for toothache are tooth decay, mouth bacteria, tooth cavity and excessive consumption of soft drinks, candies, chocolates, refined carbohydrates and sugar. Toothache can be mild, moderate, chronic or severe in nature. It can, however, be treated by resorting to the natural ways.

Home Remedy for Toothache

- Place a clove of garlic, dipped in rock salt, under the affected tooth. Alternatively, chew a clove of garlic every morning. Along with curing the teeth, it would also make them strong.

- Another effective home remedy for toothache would be to chew a raw onion everyday. It is believed that chewing a raw onion for three minutes every day is sufficient to kill all the germs in the mouth.
- Lime serves as a rich source of Vitamin C and is, thus, effective in curing all the dental problems. Rubbing a piece of lime on the aching tooth is sure to bring relief.
- Wheat grass proves beneficial in the treatment of toothache. Whenever you are suffering from the ailment, chew a piece of wheat grass. It would help in extracting the toxins from the gum and also provide relief.
- Grind some asafetida and lemon juice. Now, heat this solution slightly. Dip a cotton ball in it and place it over the tooth cavity.
- Make a paste with bay berry and vinegar. Apply this paste over the affected tooth.
- Clove oil proves useful in treating toothache. Apply this oil over the affected tooth and leave there for sometime.
- To a 1/4 tsp of common salt, add a pinch of pepper powder. Apply this mixture over the affected tooth. This is sure to relieve a person from pain.
- Add a pinch of pepper in ½ tsp of clove oil and apply on the affected tooth to get relief.
- For instant relief, put 2 to 3 drops of vanilla extract on the aching tooth.
- Another effective home remedy would be to peel a potato and cut it into slices. Put one of the slices on the aching tooth, for 15 minutes.
- Dip a tea bag in a cup of boiling water. Once the tea bag gets hot, place it over the tooth. This would provide instant relief.
- Applying oregano oil on the tooth would provide relief from the pain.

- Another effective home remedy would be to chew some leaves of the guava tree.
- Place an ice cube over the aching tooth, for about 15 to 20 minutes. Repeat the process at least three to four times a day.
- Soak a cotton ball in brandy and squeeze it over the affected tooth.
- Rinse the affected tooth with some whiskey. For this, take a mouthful of whiskey and savor it over the affected tooth for sometime.
- For toothache that results from trapped food, take a mouthful of water and rinse your mouth thoroughly. This would surely help in removing the stuck food particles.
- In 3 to 4 drops of mustard oil, add a pinch of salt. Massage the jaws with this mixture. Not only would it provide relief from toothache, but also make the gums and jaws strong.

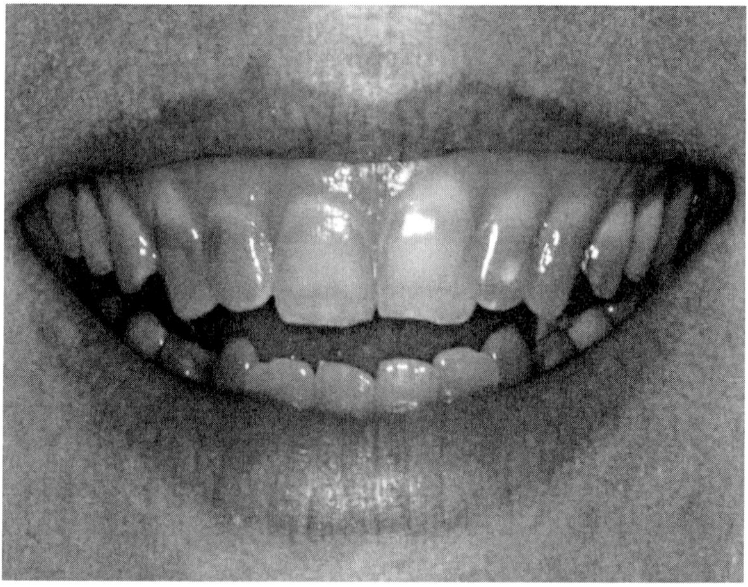

102. Discoloration of Teeth

Discoloration of teeth has become a common problem now-a-days. It affects one and all, be it men, women or children. A person requires lots of precautionary measures to retain the shinning white color of his/her teeth. Smoking, chewing of tobacco, chemotherapy, excessive fluoride use, bad eating and drinking habits, improper and irregular brushing of the teeth and diseases are some of the common causes of teeth discoloration. Its symptoms include sticky tar deposits, bad breath, tooth decay, brown tooth stains and inflammation of the roof of the mouth. Sometimes, strong medicines and genetic problems also cause teeth discoloration. It can, however, be treated at home using the natural treatments.

Home Remedy for Teeth Discoloration

- Baking soda is a very good whitening agent. You can prepare toothpaste with baking soda, lime and salt, adding a few drops of lime as well. Use it to clean your teeth on a daily basis.

- A number of fruits have bleaching properties and can help remove teeth discoloration. Include fruits like strawberries, lemon and oranges in your diet.
- Mouthwash proves beneficial in removing teeth discoloration. After having meals, make sure to rinse your mouth with a mouthwash. It does not let the stains accumulate.
- Include lots of vegetables, like cucumbers, broccoli, carrots and sweet potatoes, in your diet. They help dissolve the molecules that cause deep stains.
- You should brush the teeth regularly, at least two times in a day, to avoid discoloration of teeth.
- Rubbing the teeth with salt has been found to be effective in treating discoloration of teeth.
- After brushing your teeth, use a floss to clean the inner parts. This would help remove the food particles stuck therein, thereby curing teeth discoloration.
- Chewing sugarless gum right after meals is effective in treating discoloration of teeth.
- Avoid foods and beverages that leave a stain on the teeth. They would add to the discoloration problem.

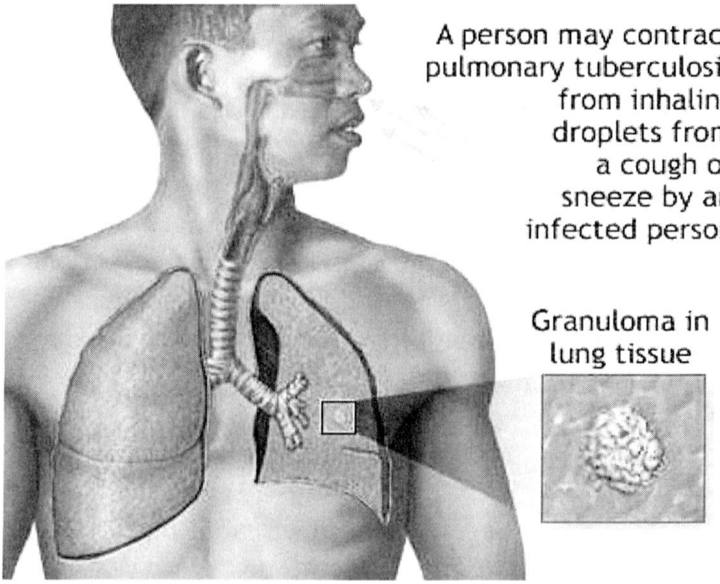

103. Tuberculosis

A infection of the lungs, Tuberculosis is caused by the bacteria Mycobacterium tuberculosis. The germ enters the body through the nose, mouth or windpipe and stays down in the tile lungs. The causes of tuberculosis include low resistance of the body, smoking, drinking and stress. The symptoms of this disease begin with cough and extend to chest pain, prolonged coughing and bringing out blood with cough. Fever, chills, sweating in the night, loss of appetite and weight loss are some other symptoms associated with tuberculosis. Though a brutal disease of the yester years, tuberculosis can now be successfully treated, even at home.

Home Remedy for Tuberculosis

- Mix 5 grams asafetida with 10 grams each of camphor and kattha and 10 tender leaves of the neem. Now, add the juice of Holy Basil leaves to this mixture, to form a paste. From the paste, make small tablets, of the size of chickpeas. Take one pellet at a time, dipped in rose essence, 3 to 4 times in a day.

- Wash and grind the leaves of celery and extract its juice. Have this juice at regular intervals of an hour. For the first time, have four tbsp of this juice and then, cut it down to 2 tbsp. Continue until the stools become rigid.
- In a bowl, mix 10 pieces each of black pepper and asafetida, fried in ghee. Add a few drops of opium to it. Now, blend them properly and make small tablets. Have one pellet, with water, after every 6 hours.
- In some clove oil, add a few pieces of crystallized sugar. Let it sit for sometime. Have this mixture several times a day.
- Nutmeg and jaggery are helpful in curing tuberculosis. Crush a nutmeg into a powdery form and add jaggery to it. When the mixture gets in a paste form, make small pellets of it, each weighing 3 milligrams. Have a pellet, with warm water, after every half an hour.
- For aches and pains, crush nutmeg to make a fine powder. Now, add 100 milliliters of oil in it and cook it on a low flame. Once warm, apply this oil on the hands and legs of the ailing person.
- In a juice of onion, add a bit of asafetida. Have this mixture every half an hour, to relieve a person of tuberculosis.
- Mix a tsp each of mint juice and honey. To this, add 2 tsp of malt vinegar. Now, add the mixture to a cupful of carrot juice and stir the liquids completely. Have this juice three times a day.
- Increase the consumption of bottle gourd, as it the best vegetable for increasing the body's resistance to tuberculosis.
- In a bowl of water, immerse some leaves of drumstick tree. Now, boil the water. Strain it and flavor with some

salt, pepper and a dash of lemon juice. Have this soup every morning, on an empty stomach.

- In a glass of orange juice, add a tbsp of honey and a pinch of salt. Have this juice everyday, on an empty stomach.
- Extract the juice of a single berry and add equal amounts of honey to it. Have this juice every morning, on an empty stomach.
- Combine some sugar candy and ghee in butter. Have this blended mixture several times a day.
- Regular consumption of pineapple juice has proved to be helpful in treating tuberculosis.
- Add some sugar to large black raisins. Now, sprinkle some black pepper over them and grind to make a powdery substance. Have a tbsp of this powder, two times a day.
- In a glass of milk, add 5 pieces of long pepper and sugar to taste. Boil the milk and allow it to get warm. Strain the milk and have it two times a day.

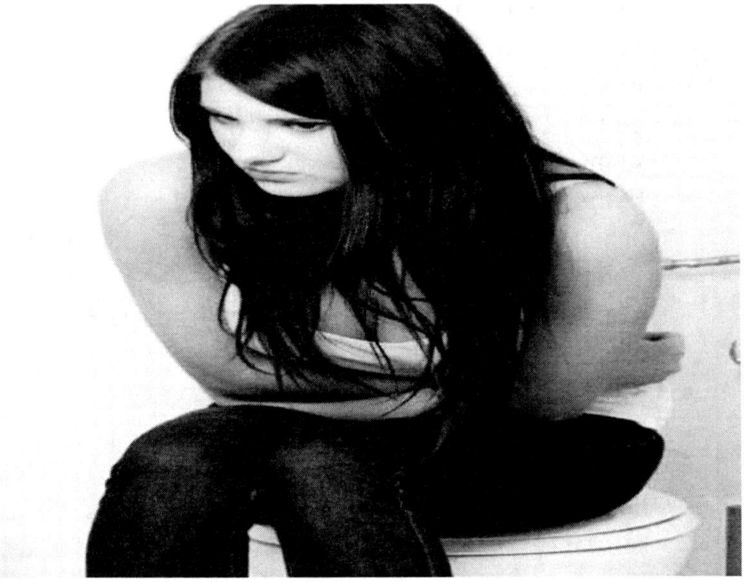

104. Urinary Tract Infection

An invasion of bacteria into the urinary tract causes UTI (Urinary Tract Infection). The bacteria enter from the opening of the urethra and proceed further into the urinary tract. Some of the causes of UTI include sexual intercourse, multiple sexual partners and holding urine for too long. Urinary tract infection can be very painful, if not treated in time. It can also spread to the kidney, causing serious health problems. Though the disease can affect members of both the sex, women are more susceptible to it. Some of the common symptoms of urinary tract infection are burning sensation while urinating, a constant urge to urinate, blood in the urine, fever, vomiting, nausea, backache and pain below the ribs.

Home Remedy for Urinary Tract Infection

- Baking soda is effective in curing urinary tract infection. In an eight ounce glass of water, add ½ tsp of baking soda. Mix this well and drink it.

- Have plenty of water in a day, as this would help in diluting and flushing out the unwanted substances from the body.
- Drinking cranberry juice is another effective way to treat urinary tract infection. For people who cannot have pure cranberry juice, mixing it with some apple juice is an option.
- Mix equal proportions of sandalwood, bergamot, tea tree, frankincense and juniper oil. Rub this combination of oil in the abdominal area once a day, for three to four days.
- Mix equal parts of pipsissewa, buchu, echinacea and urva ursi tinctures. Have 20 drops of this mixture, every two hours, for the first two days and 1 tsp of this mixture, four times a day, later on.
- Another useful remedy for UTI would be to boil the leaves of blue brinjal plant in water. Cool the decoction, strain it and have an ounce of it two times in a day.
- Boil some coriander seeds in water. Cool the decoction, strain it and have an ounce of it two times in a day. It will increase the urine flow.
- The seeds of carrot are useful in treating urinary tract infection. They can either be taken as an infusion or as a decoction.
- In a bowl of water, put some petals of lotus and pink rose and bring it to boil. Strain the liquid after it cools. Have an ounce of this, three times a day.
- Chameli plant decoction is helpful in curing urinary tract infection. In a bowl of water, put chameli plant and bring it to boil. Allow it to cool. Strain the liquid and drink it once daily.

105. Varicose Veins

Derived from a Latin word 'varix', which means twisted, varicose is a situation that arises as a result of weak veins. Veins are the carriers of impure blood, from the different parts of the body, back to the heart. When these veins become weak, instead of carrying the blood to the heart, they flow it back, thus resulting in congestion. Though the problem of varicose veins may occur in any part of the body, legs are the most susceptible region. The causes of varicose veins include pregnancy, obesity, long-standing periods and lack of exercise. Varicose veins can, however, be treated using home remedies. In the following lines, we have provided some of the ways to cure the problem at home.

Home Remedy for Varicose Veins

- One of the most effective ways of treating varicose veins would be to have a combination of carrot and spinach juice. For this, combine 300 ml of carrot juice and 200 ml of spinach juice.
- Vitamin E and C are essential for the treatment of varicose vein. For this, take 3,000 mg of vitamin C and 600 to 1,200 mg of vitamin E daily.

- Staying on an all-fruit diet, for two to three days, is an easy solution for varicose veins. Thereafter, have a balanced diet that includes grains, seeds, nuts, raw vegetables and fresh fruits.
- Warm water enema is a good home remedy to cure varicose veins, as it helps cleanse the bowels.
- Applying apple cider vinegar to the varicose veins two times a day i.e. in the morning and evening would prove helpful in treating the problem. This would make the vein shrink back to their original size.
- Taking hot Epsom salt bath, two times in a week, will prove effective in treating varicose veins.
- Another useful home remedy would be to massage the affected area with rosemary oil.
- Take some fuller's earth powder and add some water to it, until it forms a paste. Apply this mudpack on the affected area at night and leave it on till the morning. Then, rinse off with water.
- In 4 ounces of carrier oil (almond oil), add 12 drops each of cypress and rosemary essential oils. Apply this mixture on the legs, by gently stroking them in an upward motion. This is an effective way to treat varicose veins.
- Applying vitamin E oil or witch hazel tea to the affected area serves as a good home remedy for varicose veins.
- Take hot and cold hip bath, alternately. This would prove to be beneficial in curing varicose veins.
- Mix together 2 cups each of chopped calendula flowers, leaves and stems, along with melted lard. After about 24 hours, heat the mixture and strain it. Apply this over the varicose veins.
- Avoid having potatoes, starchy foods, condiments, alcohol, coffee, strong tea, white flour products and white sugar, when suffering from varicose veins.

106. Vomiting

An ejection of food and liquids from the stomach, through the contraction of the stomach muscle, is called vomiting. Also known as emesis, vomiting leads to the expulsion of solids as well as liquids, from the stomach. There are many reasons for vomiting like overeating, drinking excessive alcohol, pregnancy, migraine, infections, flu, upset stomach, etc. At times, vomiting is also one of the symptoms for a major disease as well. Its own symptoms include increased saliva, dizziness, light-headedness, difficulty in swallowing food or liquid, changes in skin temperature and increase in the rate of heartbeat.

Home Remedy for Vomiting

- One of the effective ways to cure vomiting would be to have ginger tea. Make sure it has less amount of sugar.
- Chilled lime juice also proves effective in treating vomiting. In a glass of cold water, squeeze 1 lime. Add sugar and salt to taste. Put in some ice, to chill it. Drink this mixture after every two hours.
- If the vomiting is due to excess intake of alcohol, eat a slice or two of bread slowly, so that it soaks the liquid.
- Do not eat any solid food until after 12 hours of vomiting. Instead, have loads of vegetable juices, water and other

non-acid drinks. Then only, start having solid foods, such as mashed potatoes, rice and oatmeal.

- On a non-stick pan, heat 2 cardamoms. Once heated, crush them to form a powder and add a tsp of honey to it. Have this several times a day.
- Prepare a mixture by combining 1 tsp each of mint juice and lime juice, with 1/2 tsp ginger juice and a tsp honey. Have it 2-3 times in a day.
- Boil a cup of water and add a tsp of cinnamon or one cinnamon stick to it. Steep it for sometime and strain the water. Now, add a tbsp of honey, for sweetening it. Have this decoction 2-3 times in a day.
- Holy Basil, catnip and peach bark tea are helpful for treating vomiting. You can have them in any form you like.
- A tsp of onion juice, taken after every two hours, proves beneficial in curing vomiting.
- Mix ¼ tsp powdered ginger, 1 cup apple juice and ¼ cup water together. Blend the mixture well, until the ginger gets dissolved, and add enough ice to make it slushy.
- Mix 1 tbsp each of apple cider vinegar and honey in a glass of normal water and drink it before going to bed.
- Put some cloves, cardamoms or a cinnamon stick in your mouth. This is an effective way to treat vomiting.
- Cut a lemon into two halves. Sprinkle some rock salt on one of its piece. Lick this piece till all the juice runs out.
- Boil ½ cup of rice in 1 to 1½ cup of water. When the rice gets cooked, strain the water and drink it. It will help cease vomiting.
- Intaking half a tsp of grounded cumin seeds, along with water, is helpful in stopping vomiting.
- Avoid too much of oily, spicy food, heavy and indigestible food, when you are suffering from vomiting.

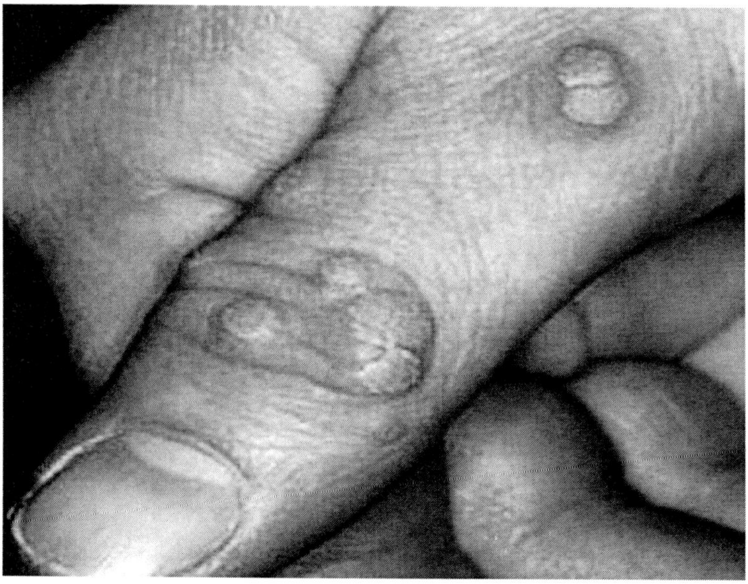

107. Warts

Warts have become a common problem among adults as well as children. Classified within the Human Papilloma Viruses, though harmless, warts have the capability of spreading to all the parts of the body. They can occur anywhere - skin, mouth, genitals, rectal area, etc. Also referred to as skin tumors, they can be classified into various types, such as common warts, foot warts, flat warts and genital warts. Warts appear as rough elevations on the skin, generally on the fingers, elbows, knees, face and scalp. Primarily caused by virus infection, warts can also result from defects in the proper development of skin surface, in certain areas. Warts can, however, be treated using home remedies.

Home Remedy for Warts

- A poultice of flaxseed is beneficial in treating warts. For this, mix ground flaxseeds with flaxseed oil and add a small quantity of raw honey. Apply this on the wart and cover with a bandage. Prepare a fresh poultice everyday.
- Another effective remedy would be to crush a clove of garlic and apply it on the affected area. Now, cover it with a bandage.

- Applying freshly cut pineapple over the affected area, several times a day, is an effective way of curing warts.
- Extract the juice of fig stems and apply this over the affected area. It is a good way to treat warts.
- Squeeze the white milky juice from a dandelion weed. Put this juice over the warts, for removing them.
- Camphor oil proves effective in removing warts. Coat the affected area with camphor oil, several times in a day.
- Massaging the affected area with castor oil, two times a day, would make it soft and free of warts
- Extract grapefruit juice and apply a drop or two on the affected area, 3 to 4 times in a day. Cover the area with a cloth or a bandage.
- Applying tea tree oil on the affected area will prove helpful in removing the warts.
- Soak the area with warm water, for about 15 to 20 minutes. Thereafter, apply cider vinegar, with cotton balls, and leave it to dry. Now, wash the area with plain water and pat it dry.
- Peel a banana and tape its peel over the wart, with the inner side on top of the infection. Change the peel every 12 to 24 hours.
- Soak a slice of onion in vinegar overnight. In the morning, place the soaked piece over the affected area and bandage it.
- Apply powder of herb Indian squill over the warts, on a daily basis.
- Rubbing a piece of chalk or raw potato on the affected area. This will help remove the warts.
- Apply the oil extracted from the shell of the cashew nut over the warts and bandage the area.

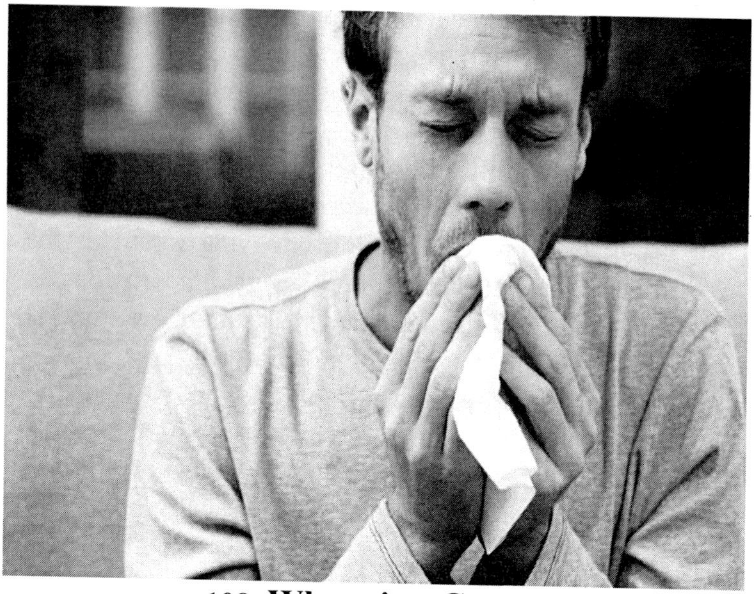

108. Whooping Cough

The bacterial infection in lungs, caused by bacterium Bordetella pertussis, is called whooping cough. A contagious disease, it leads to severe coughing, which may or may not be accompanied by vomiting and perspiration. Some of the common symptoms of whooping cough are sore throat, mild dry cough, sneezing, tears, tiredness, loss of appetite, night cough, vomiting, retching, nosebleeds and diarrhea. Though it starts with a mild cough, whooping cough develops into severe coughing, if not treated on time. Whooping cough can, however, be treated with home remedies as well.

Home Remedy for Whooping Cough

- One of most effective home remedies for whooping cough would be to have a cup of grape juice, mixed with a tsp of honey, on a daily basis.
- Soak 7 almonds in water, overnight. In the morning, remove the brown skin and pound the almonds, to form a paste. Now, add 20 grams each of butter and sugar.

Consume the paste two times a day, in the morning and evening.

- Finely chop an onion and extract its juice. Mix 1 tsp of this juice with 1 tsp of honey and keep it aside. Consume it after four to five hours.
- Crush a medium-sized onion and add the juice of one lemon to it. Now, pour a cup of boiling water over it and add a tsp of honey. Take this 2 to 3 times a day.
- Roast and powder the root of turmeric. Take 3 grams of this powder, along with milk, two times a day.
- Mix 2 grams of the pulp of the herb of belleric myroblan, 1/4 tsp salt, 1/2 tsp long pepper and 2 tsp honey. Have this mixture two times a day.
- Dry the herb of belleric myroblan and cover it with wheat flour. Now, roast the herb and consume it.
- Grind 100 gm of raisins, with water. Add 100 gm of sugar to the paste. Once it forms a saucy consistency, preserve it. Have 20 grams of this mixture everyday, before going to bed.
- Aniseed is helpful in treating whooping cough. Prepare a tea with it and have it 1-2 times in a day.
- Extract garlic juice and have a tsp of this, 2 to 3 times a day. This is an effective way to treat whooping cough.
- In a cup of water, add a tsp each of fenugreek seeds and fresh ginger, along with a dash of honey. Bring the water to a boil and allow it to cool. Strain the drink and consume it.
- Mix 5-6 drops of almond oil and 10 drops each of ginger juice and onion oil. Have this mixture three times daily.
- Cut a small slice of ginger and dip it in some rock salt and lemon juice. Store this in an airtight container. Lick this whenever the cough attacks.

- Mix a tsp of fresh radish juice with equal quantity of honey. Add some rock salt and form syrup. Consume this every 8 hours.
- Take a tbsp of carrot juice, mixed with some honey and warm water. This proves beneficial in treating whooping cough.

□□□